SILENT TRAUMA

THE SIDE OF HEALTHCARE WE DON'T TALK ABOUT

BRIAN W. WILLIAMSON

RN, CEN, CCRN, CRFN, CLNC

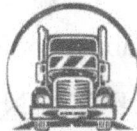

BABTS PUBLISHING

Published in 2025 by BADTS Publishing

Ebook ISBN: 979-8-9932679-0-6
Paperback ISBN: 979-8-9932679-1-3
Hardcover ISBN: 979-809932679-2-0
Audiobook ISBN: 979-8-9932679-3-7

Printed in the United States of America

Book cover design by Bekah Ott
Technical edits by Paul Tabladillo, RN, MSN-Ed, AG-ACNP BC, PHN
Image subject: Sheila Anulao, RN, MSN-Ed, CEN, CPEN

To my all-time greatest mentor, whom I approached hundreds of times with life's challenges. His response to me was always the same:

"I don't have to live with your choices; you do. What do you think you should do?"

I think he'd like this book. I miss him every day.

I Love You, Pop

FOREWORD

If you work in the emergency room or are a first responder, you know the reality of seeing things nobody should ever have to see. Then what do you do? You maintain composure while dealing with human tragedy, give horrible news to sobbing family members, clean the blood off our shoes, and walk into the next room with a smile—because that's what is expected of us.

In this book, Brian finally sheds light on what happens to *us*. He does this not only to ignite change in the industry but also to help our families understand a little bit better what we go through and why we are the way we are.

Brian doesn't sugarcoat it—he pulls back the curtain on a reality many of us know but few are ever able to fully process as we continue working on the front lines of life and death. The truth is, trauma is part of the job, and we've been taught—or expected—to suck it up and move on.

I vividly recall my first call as a firefighter paramedic. It was the late 1980s, and we responded to a vehicle rollover involving a student from the local university. As the medic, it was my job to gain entry to the vehicle and perform an assessment. This was the first time I smelled blood, brain, and twisted metal within the confines of a compact vehicle. What did we do after determining the life of a beautiful eighteen-year-old female had been tragically cut short? We went right back to the station to await the next call. In those days, we did not even clean our turnouts or change into a second set after a call. Dirty turnouts—blood and soot—were a badge of honor of sorts. The average first responder or healthcare professional will encounter hundreds of such scenarios during their career. The majority of those scenarios will not be followed by a debrief.

I am proud of my colleagues in this profession. They are some of the most resilient people on the planet. Resilience makes them remarkably good at this difficult job. That resilience also comes at a cost.

We are humans first, and our trauma inevitably starts to show up in our personal and sometimes even our professional lives. This often looks like risky or daredevil behavior, dark humor, anxiety, burnout, strained relationships, exhaustion, sleep deprivation, or all of the above. Within our field, everyone knows this is a struggle, but where is the support for acknowledging and processing our trauma?

This important book takes you through several heart-wrenching, real-life stories Brian and other healthcare professionals have experienced. It outlines the very real trauma experienced in our line of work and the lack of support we receive when the dust settles.

Brian is the ideal voice to speak on this subject. With decades of experience as a critical care nurse, an emergency department nurse, and a flight nurse, he has had a front-row seat to the most difficult moments in healthcare. His insight is grounded not only in clinical expertise but also in the deep emotional toll that comes with giving exceptional care to his patients in the most heartbreaking moments. I've witnessed him do this many times, proudly calling him a partner and colleague.

Brian is providing a platform to discuss the solutions and trauma support we desperately need. For healthcare workers, having a stronger support system is as critical to survival as the life-and-death care we provide our patients.

Jacqueline C. Stocking, PhD, MBA, MSN, NEA-BC, CMTE, CEN, CFRN, FP-C, CCP-C, RN, NRP, FAASTN

Vice Chair – Quality and Safety - University of California, Davis

PREFACE

A fifty-three-year-old wife and mother of four sits in the closet of her bedroom with the door closed. She has a glass of wine and a handful of various pills. She thinks of her children and husband. Of how wonderful they are and how full of excitement for Thanksgiving, a week away. She wonders who will find her and what state she will be in. Will she have vomited? Will she have soiled herself? Will they mourn for a long time? Will her husband remarry? Will she suffer, or will she just fall asleep forever?

A fifty-nine-year-old father and grandfather finishes his day at work. He bids his colleagues' good night and tells them he will see them in the morning. Everything seems great. He leaves work in his pickup truck and heads out of town. He thinks of his grandson and the fishing trip they are planning for the weekend. He thinks of his wonderful wife of thirty-five years. He parks his truck under a tree off the main road. He calls 911 to let them know where they can find his body, then hangs up and takes his handgun from the glove compartment.

A twenty-eight-year-old single woman is working her dream job she worked for years to get, a job for which she was willing to relocate in order to have the best opportunity. She is a stellar employee. She manages all her duties flawlessly. Her coworkers and those she encounters daily love her demeanor. Inside, however, she is feeling overwhelmed by her job. She has been feeling this way for months. She has thought about suicide and has even formulated a plan. One day while working, she breaks. Nothing unusual or out of the ordinary happened at work, but she breaks anyway. She leaves the building to go outside and cry. An observant coworker follows her. She tells her coworker everything, including that she is seriously considering suicide. Her coworker intervenes and gets her to the emergency room, where she is evaluated and admitted to the mental health unit for treatment.

None of the individuals mentioned in these scenarios had a history of mental illness. None were on any medications. They all had normal upbringings and are educated professionals. They had different backgrounds, and all had supportive, solid families. So, what do they all have in common besides the real desire to end their own lives?

They are all part of a profession that exposes them to stressors most people cannot even imagine. A profession equipped to deal with the kind of mental stress these individuals experience. However, the profession is not focused on these individuals. It is not a profession where the leadership expects them to be affected. In fact, in most cases, the members of leadership in this profession are often surprised by the profound effect of stress on their employees and are unprepared to effectively deal with it.

It may surprise most people to know these individuals are all registered nurses. They are healers, nurturers, and angels of mercy. According to polls, they are the most trusted of all professionals worldwide. These are the professionals everyday people turn to when they need care from physical, psychological, and emotional turmoil. How, then, is it possible for these caregivers to fall prey to the very tragedies they spend their entire careers helping others face?

Most people today have heard of post-traumatic stress disorder (PTSD). This is something most often associated with the military. As mental health has evolved and the exposure that contributes directly to PTSD has been identified and defined, it has become clear the members of the armed forces in combat roles are not alone in this sometimes debilitating disorder.

Recent findings show registered nurses commit suicide at a rate of 23.8 per 100,000—18% higher than the general population (20.1 per 100,000). Among female nurses, the rate is nearly double: 17.1 versus 8.6 per 100,000. (Davis et al. 2021)

When the focus is on emergency services, which includes EMTs, paramedics, firefighters, law enforcement, and medical flight teams, the rates are significantly higher. Nearly half (46.8%) of firefighters report suicidal ideation, nearly one in five (19.2%) report forming a plan, and almost one in six (15.5%) report an actual suicide attempt during their career. (Vigil et al. 2021)

I have often said that everyone in my business is affected by what we see. Those who say they are not affected are either being dishonest, do not understand what constitutes being affected, or are sociopaths. You cannot do what we do and see what we see, day in and day out, without being affected. Of course, in time, we all build up lines of defense within ourselves to help set our experiences in a corner of our minds enough to allow us to function in our respective roles. However, we *are* all affected. And we all need to detox from what we experience in this business.

I believe there is a scale we are all on in dealing with our experience. On one end, there are people who seem to be dealing with things just fine. They might have strong faith and spouses, families, or groups of friends who help them remain grounded by allowing them to detox emotionally. Some have a pet, do yoga, exercise, hike, or get out in the wilderness. Then, there are those who either do not have these or are not effectively using their resources to detox. These people may drink, become promiscuous, abuse their families, or become addicted to substances. Some just change professions and get away from it. Some engage in extremely risky physical behavior. On the other end of the scale, there are those who attempt or commit suicide. Of course, there are scores of items that could be added to this scale, as I have just listed a few. But I do believe we all need to detox in our own way because we *are* all affected.

This book will address what I believe are some of the stressors people working in emergency healthcare come in contact with every day, as well as the reasons this stress goes unreported and unaddressed. Responses from colleagues and organizational leadership will also be addressed. I will do this from the perspective and experience of working for four decades in the trenches of direct patient contact in the world of emergency care. My personal experiences come from my days as a young EMT in northern Los Angeles County, a registered nurse in the ICU and emergency rooms of Southern California, and as a flight nurse in Southern California. However, this applies to healthcare workers in and out of the hospital: EMS workers, law enforcement, and firefighters. I will be using personal experiences to help me convey the emotional side of what we do. However, each person in my profession could exchange their own experiences with mine. Mine are no more profound than those of my colleagues. They just happen to be the ones I have firsthand knowledge of. Nearly all the examples I use in this book are real experiences. I do my best to relay them as accurately as possible.

Some of the examples I use will illustrate what I believe contributes to the stress experienced in healthcare. Some are acts of commission, and others omission, by frontline workers, supervisors, and hospital administration. Though my examples are specific, they represent a culture that exists in the industry as a whole. I use specific examples to bring credibility to my message. Speaking in general terms often creates a more arguable climate, where the audience is left to decide what the author is referring to. By using specifics, I hope to bring the reader along for a firsthand glimpse into the world of emergency healthcare workers and the experiences affecting them, and the toxic culture that has become the norm. My intent is not to paint any individual or organization in a negative light. I try to avoid identifying organizations or individuals that contribute to this toxicity, intentionally or otherwise. I believe the culture is global. There will also be those who read this and have worked in an area where this toxic culture is minimized by quality support and intervention. There are exceptions to my overall conclusions. However, those great examples are anecdotal and should be considered examples of what the industry *should* be doing.

As I began working on this book, I assumed my audience would be my colleagues. That is, those people who work in the emergency room and emergency services outside the hospital. I have come to realize a larger audience—family members and close friends of my colleagues and me. Many family members see stress on our faces. They try to help when we have had a bad day. They ask questions and sincerely want to know what they can do. The problem? Most people who work in emergency services are very good at protecting loved ones from the horrors they keep in their heads and only talk about difficult cases and situations, generally. Still, they do not share the details of how these experiences affect them and make them feel.

Many who read this do not have clinical roles in healthcare; instead, they are colleagues who work beside nurses and doctors, but who are not medical clinicians. In the ER, there are secretaries, registration clerks, housekeepers, security, social workers, etc., experiencing the chaos and tragedy as well. Because of this, I try to speak in lay terms as much as possible. Some of my clinical peeps may wonder why I am explaining things that may seem very basic to us. It is for those who work with us and are not clinical, as well as those who are family members and friends outside the industry. When telling stories, unless I state otherwise, I use the real names of those involved. I do this to help readers realize these are not statistics. They are people.

I hope this book will help my colleagues realize it is okay to acknowledge the stress we feel and reach out for help when needed. However, my broader goal is for all who work in emergency services and acute healthcare to be aware of signs in those they work with. Additionally, I want family members and close friends of emergency service workers to be able to recognize these signs and have a deeper understanding of what their loved ones experience while at work. Sometimes, others will see stress in us before we recognize it in ourselves.

I hope this book sheds light on the things those in my profession spend so much time trying to hide from our loved ones—or simply hide from. Those closest to us need to understand the side of us they have never really seen. Not the gruesome details, but the burden we carry from these experiences. This will help them know what it is we keep bottled up and how to help us when we try so hard to deny we ever need any help at all.

Side note: The three examples used at the beginning of this preface are real. None of the individuals followed through with their plans of suicide.

INTRODUCTION

There are many stressors we face in life. Some are universal to everyone, such as family, financial concerns, running a home, interactions with friends, illness, and the like. Healthcare workers do not hold a corner of the market on stressors.

Over the years, I have heard many complaints from colleagues about their jobs and the general way they feel they are viewed by administration. Early in my career, I wondered why there was so much complaining; even now, I continue to hear things like, "This hospital should be grateful I keep coming to work here." I see so many stressed out from the time they clock in at the beginning of their shift. Of course, many others seem to be happy, no matter what comes their way. In my early days, working in the emergency room, I do not remember people complaining about how they felt stuck. Perhaps this was because I worked in the northernmost part of Los Angeles County, and there was tremendous longevity in our hospital. We had a terrific department director, Linda Lawson, who came up through the ranks. She was one of the emergency room staff nurses I admired and looked up to, when I was a young emergency medical technician (EMT) working on the ambulance. I learned much from her and the other nurses in that ER.

I was not a brand-new nurse when I came to work in the ER. When I entered the profession, there was no shortage of nurses as there is today. I wanted to work in that ER from the time I started taking classes to get into a nursing program. I naively thought a nurse's job was not much different than mine as an EMT. I remember thinking I needed to get my nursing license so I could finally get paid for the job I was already doing—essentially the same job the nurses were doing. Knowing now how ridiculous my thinking was makes me embarrassed to even mention it.

Once I was licensed, I was informed the ER was a department new graduate nurses never worked in. It was unheard of, at least in my community. Moreover, not only did registered nurses have to be experienced to work in the ER, but they had to have critical care experience. It could be adult, pediatric, or neonatal, but it had to be a critical care setting. I argued that I had been an EMT and ER tech. I knew I was someone who could do the job without going to the ICU first. However, there were no exceptions. So, I went kicking and screaming to the ICU because I had to. In retrospect, I am so thankful for the strict position Linda took. I would have never known what I did not know about critical care nursing without that experience.

I quickly realized how different things were as an ER nurse, compared to the intensive care unit. It helped having a great department director. If I had a question or screwed something up, Linda never made me feel stupid. When I needed counseling on something, I never felt picked on or attacked. To me, it seemed as if I had the perfect job in the perfect hospital with the perfect boss and the perfect group of individuals to work with and mentor me. Those nurses, techs, and doctors taught me much more than ER medicine and allowed me to be able to capitalize on the opportunities I have had throughout my career. I will be forever thankful to them for getting me started on the path that has brought me to where I am today.

I went into nursing because I had been involved in healthcare since I was sixteen. My first real job was delivering oxygen for the local ambulance company in town. I thought it was so cool to watch one of my best friends, Doug McCullough, blast down the road with sirens blaring. I signed up for the EMT program when I was seventeen. I was moved from delivering oxygen to working on the ambulance, just before my eighteenth birthday. I had the coolest

3

job at a small private company, Wilson Ambulance. I loved being an EMT, but the pay was terrible at that time. After getting married, I tried several different things. I did retail, automotive service and product sales, construction, and several other things, but I continued working on the weekends as an EMT.

I eventually opted to work toward becoming a nurse, but I did not choose nursing for the same reasons many other people do, like wanting to care for people. I did not have an experience with a loved one being cared for by wonderful nurses. I did not have a kind, caring heart or want to give back. I did, however, enjoy working in emergency services. It was something many people have said, "I could never do that." I liked that I could do what others said they could not, and I knew it paid way better than being an EMT. So my reasoning was strictly practical and a bit arrogant. I wanted a job in high demand that I already had some familiarity with and something not everyone could do. It was also a recession-proof job. No matter what the economy was like, I would always have a job.

With all of that, I ended up with a good job and steady pay. As a boy, I always saw my parents work hard. I was taught by my father to be thankful I had an opportunity to provide for my family. Pop had a job outside the home, and he worked very hard. He seemed to always be awake—most of the time already gone when I got up and awake when I went to bed. Except for occasional naps in the chair on a Sunday afternoon, I wondered if he ever slept. He worked some Saturdays and would take my siblings and me with him. I never once heard him complain. Mom was a full-time homemaker. She worked tirelessly to take care of the house, seven kids, Pop, and actively participated in all our activities. She, too, was up before me and after I went to bed. I am sure they complained to each other about being overwhelmed at times. However, they set a great example of not complaining about hard work.

As an adult, I came to realize life's stressors. I have had my ups and downs like everybody else. Still, it seems people in my profession, especially emergency services, have a unique ability to be stressed more than others. I have been frustrated to hear nurses talk about how hard the job is and how nobody understands. Not because I do not believe their sincerity, but because it is a terrific profession. I have always understood we deal with people's lives and tragedies. However, in every profession, some feel underpaid, underappreciated, overworked, and overwhelmed. Still, there is something strange going on in my profession I have come to realize is a poison, a toxic culture affecting all of us and causing many to flee from patient care. Stressors of life, along with the generally accepted stress of healthcare, are certainly factors, but there is something else I have found is strangely unique to emergency services, which I will attempt to identify. Specifically, I will try to explain the more unique culture that seems to fester within emergency services. I will also share a small part of my journey in realizing the unspoken stressors creating and perpetuating a toxic culture.

FACING THE STRESS

There are many different things we stress over. Not all are specific to the medical field, but there are some that are unique to my profession.

The first and most obvious type involves direct patient contact. This comes in the form of a tragic event, which alone can be immediately and emotionally disruptive to those involved. All who go into healthcare know they will encounter tragedy. We read newspapers and books or watch the news and movies where bad things happen to people, then medical professionals get involved. Some have experienced human tragedy firsthand. Still, those who enter healthcare do not understand what they have gotten into until they are already committed to their careers. That is, working with strangers, often during the worst time of their lives

From the very beginning of our education and training, we learn to get into other people's personal space. At its basic level, this is the first big hurdle to overcome when working in healthcare. Over time, we become very comfortable being up close and personal with strangers. However, we all have a moment in our career where we are forced to face the reality of what real human tragedy is. Some will go many months or years before encountering such a situation. But regardless of how long it takes, the day will come when we are faced with the reality of the profession we have chosen and the devastation that happens to ordinary people every day. Additionally, we begin to understand this type of situation is not a one-off. It happens again and again! I have interviewed hundreds of colleagues for this book, and without exception, whoever I am speaking with will say something like, "I remember this one time . . ." Then, they would recount, with some emotion, a situation where the circumstances were so intense, they burned the details of that situation into their mind. We *all* have one of those times. Given enough time in this business, most of us will have many!

The Baby

As a young eighteen-year-old EMT, I thought I had the world by the tail. It was 1984. I had keys to an expensive ambulance—a Ford high-top ambulance with a big block 460, covered in chrome and red lights with sirens so loud they would drown out any sound. I was cool! My buddies were working in fast food, in a warehouse, in an office, in the military, or they were in college. What sunglasses looked the coolest was my primary worry. I had been on the job less than four months, but I had grown up in this town and knew it like the back of my hand. The problem: I was young, inexperienced, immature, and, most importantly, did not know it.

My partner and I were out driving in town when a call came in for a sick child. Because we were already out, we were the closest basic life support (BLS) ambulance to the address and were dispatched, along with the fire department paramedics. When we pulled up in front of the house, there was a sheriff patrol car parked in front and, as expected, no other EMS personnel. We were first!

My partner was driving and pulled up to the curb. I jumped out and headed straight for the house like a boss! I thought to myself, "I've got this. I am here to save the day." As I approached the front of the house with the confidence that usually goes along with ignorance, a deputy sheriff came running out of the house with a naked infant boy in his arms. I can remember seeing the little limp body as if it were yesterday. The deputy ran straight to me and practically threw the child into my arms. I looked down at this seemingly lifeless little boy and froze. I could not think of anything to do. I was terrified. In the blink of an eye, I went from feeling like I was there to save the day to wishing I was home at my parents' house, hiding behind my mother.

After what felt like an eternity, I turned and headed for the ambulance. My partner had opened the door, and I climbed in and placed the infant on the gurney. His skin was hot. Very hot! He had a high fever. As I quickly looked at him and tried to think what to do, I noticed he was breathing. It was extremely fast and shallow, but he was breathing. My own heart was beating so hard, I thought my head would explode. At that moment, an experienced fire department paramedic climbed into the back of the ambulance and said, "Let's go!"

I had never been so happy to see someone in my entire life. My partner jumped into the front seat and stomped on the throttle. I do not remember much of the ride to the hospital, however, I do remember we began CPR before arriving at the ER. This was the first time I had ever done CPR on a real person, and it was an infant. We arrived at the ER pretty quickly, and once inside, I watched the emergency room nurses, respiratory therapist, techs, and doctor work furiously to save this little boy's life. Ultimately, they were not successful.

I remember going outside to the ambulance bay. My confidence was gone. The thrill of my job had just completely evaporated. I stood outside for a long time just thinking about that little boy. I had never experienced anything like that. After a time, my partner came outside and asked me if I was all right. I told him I did not think I could do this job. I will be forever thankful to him for his words. They were something like this: "Brian, this kind of thing sucks. But this is what the job is." We chatted for a while, and he offered some other words of encouragement and advice. I guess he got through to me because I am still in it! However, that incident has stayed with me. It rocked me, but I am still here.

This was my first lesson, though I did not realize it at the time, about how those of us who work in this industry are expected to just "shake it off" and get back to work. I talked with my family in general terms about this incident. I did not share how upset it made me. It was never discussed again at my job. I doubt anyone but my partner and I even knew what happened.

The hospital had amazing resources for the family. The child had been with a babysitter, who was brought to the hospital by the sheriff's deputy. When the parents arrived, they were all met by a very compassionate team, which included a chaplain and social worker who were trained to deal with this. They attended to the family and made sure they were comforted. They were so tender with these people and helped them through the beginning stages of this tragedy. The nurses, techs, and doctor? Well, they went back to work. So did we.

No debriefing.
No offer of assistance.

It would be easy to argue the effect this had on me was due to my inexperience and naivete in the business. That would certainly be reasonable, as our experiences, over time, help to develop our ability to better process tragedy. However, if that were entirely the case, there would be no reason to discuss this further. The fact is, we continue to be affected by human tragedy throughout our careers. As we experience more events, it seems to usually take more to get to us. Our brains also learn how to process tragedy, so we are able to function in our roles in the moment. But we are still affected by the things we see, even when we are deep into our careers and think we have "seen it all." Sometimes, even the most seasoned first responders find themselves in a situation where they are overwhelmed by the gravity of what they are experiencing.

By the time I was working as a flight nurse, I had become a seasoned professional with almost two decades under my belt in the world of emergencies. At different stages of our lives and careers, we are affected by events that mirror our own situations. We empathize with patients and families based on how their lives compare to our own. When I was young, I saw many patients as I would my own siblings or parents. Later, I would empathize as a parent and, eventually, a grandparent. This is a natural evolution and something that makes each situation unique to the caregiver involved. A team of ten people can be involved in the same incident, and yet all will be affected differently, depending on how they associate the situation with their own experience and present circumstances.

Father's Day

It was a Friday to Saturday 24-hour shift on the helicopter. We were awakened by the phone in the early hours of Saturday morning, around 3am. We were dispatched to a motor vehicle accident on a remote stretch of highway in the California desert. It was Father's Day weekend, and many people were traveling through the area headed to various recreational locations. This accident involved one of those vehicles.

A family of six was headed through our response area, in Eastern Kern County, CA, toward Lake Powell along the Utah–Arizona state line. They were in a Dodge Durango pulling a ski boat behind them. As they were motoring down the highway, they approached a rest area. At the same time, a big rig truck was exiting. For some reason, the big truck was not in much of a hurry to get up to highway speed. It was estimated by the highway patrol, the truck was traveling less than 20 mph when it entered the highway. The Durango was bearing down on the same spot at an estimated 80 mph. It was assumed the driver of the Durango must have been dozing off as he, reportedly, did not even attempt to brake when he reached the truck.

All semitrailers in the United States are required to have a T-bar on the back, which hangs down and is designed to prevent vehicles from going underneath if they hit it from the rear. When the Durango hit the back of this trailer, the T-bar failed, and the vehicle went underneath and struck the back axle. The bottom of the big rig trailer was at shoulder level of the driver, and the back of the big trailer ended up in the back seat of the Durango. The father, who was driving, was killed instantly, having been mostly decapitated. The front tip of the boat entered the back of the Durango and was impaled into the back of the truck trailer. This was a violent impact.

When we arrived on scene, the freeway was shut down. We landed our helicopter in front of the big truck. As I walked around to the passenger side of the Durango, I could see the front passenger door open and a woman sitting there. The truck trailer was where her head should be, but there were firemen working on her. I was puzzled since it appeared she was deceased. Then, her arms began moving, and I could hear her talking. It turns out that she had been leaning back asleep, and her head was tilted back, so it only appeared she was headless. She was pretty well stuck. I spoke with her and received a report from the ground paramedic. She was trapped, but her vital signs were stable, and she was oriented.

I proceeded to the back seat, where other medics were. The first thing I noticed was a young girl in the middle seat. She was six, the same age as my youngest daughter. Her head was resting against her father's. She was facing away from him and could not tell he was deceased. However, the picture of it touched me. I could not help wondering if she was comforted knowing he was there, yet having no idea he really was not. Tears welled up in my eyes for this little girl. The medic told me she would be out of the vehicle soon, and the other children were already in a triage area behind the boat trailer.

When I got to the triage spot, I noticed three additional children. It turns out they were all the same ages as my other children. I tried to stay focused, but my heart suddenly ached. As a father, it is my job to comfort my children when they are afraid. These children likely wished their father were there. They may have wondered where he and their mother were. The mother had spoken to them and told them she was okay and not to be afraid while they were still in the car. Now they were out of the vehicle and could not hear her. As I tried to focus on my job, my mind raced as I wondered how they would find out their daddy was gone. I could not help but wonder how my own children would react if it were them losing me.

Fortunately, none of the injuries the children had were life-threatening. In short order, the youngest little girl was brought to the triage area. I, along with my partner and another medic, established precautionary IVs in all the kids after assessing them and securing their spines. I was caring for the youngest little girl. She was frightened, and I did my best to comfort her. Fortunately, I was able to get an IV established quickly with only one poke.

The mother was the most seriously injured and normally would be our priority. However, she was still trapped. Since she was medically stable and did not require the advanced level of care we provided, beyond ground paramedics, I made the decision to remain with the children. We requested a second helicopter for her and decided to take all four kids with us. We operated large helicopters, and loading all four kids on our two gurneys was no problem. I spoke with the mother and assured her the kids were all okay with what appeared to be minor injuries.

I spent the majority of the forty-five-minute flight to the trauma center trying to settle the youngest child down. She was terrified by the traumatic incident. Now she was in a very dark, noisy helicopter. I had to get my mouth close to her ear and then yell for her to hear me. It was not ideal. Upon arrival at the trauma center, several of the ER staff met us on the rooftop helipad. We began offloading the children. As we moved the youngest little girl onto one of the hospital gurneys, her IV got caught on the belt of a security guard who was helping. The IV was pulled out of her arm. I just held the spot with my finger to stop the bleeding as we rode the elevator down to the trauma suite.

Once inside, there was a new experience for these kids—a very bright and busy room full of staff there to greet us. This was an academic hospital, so there were full-time healthcare professionals, as well as resident physicians and medical students. These kids were overwhelmed. The staff efficiently moved the kids into position to begin assessing them. In the ER, we often move so quickly in situations like this, we forget how scary it is for the patient. This is especially traumatic when they are young children.

In a trauma, there are people all around the patient doing different tasks. It is difficult for an adult to hear all the instructions from people around them, let alone children. "Take a deep breath," from the X-ray tech. "Are you allergic to anything?" from someone. "Where are you hurting?" from someone else. In most trauma center cases, it is well choreographed, and one person is talking to the patient at a time. However, with a multiple-casualty incident like this, the chaos is hard to avoid.

At some point, one of the nurses poked the little girl in the arm to establish a new IV. At that moment, the little girl screamed at the top of her lungs, "I want my daddy!" That was my breaking point. I had to walk away because all I could hear was my own little girl calling for me in vain to rescue her. That all the kids were the same ages as mine, they were in a hospital without their mother, they were soon to find out their daddy was dead—all of this on Father's Day weekend—was emotionally overwhelming. As I sit here writing this story, some twenty years later, I am brought to tears at the thought of it.

When we finished the call, we went back to work.

No debriefing.
No offer of assistance.

The previous example is included to illustrate the variety of situations that affect us. The father was deceased from the accident, and I never saw his injuries or dealt with him. I actually dealt with four patients, all with varying minor injuries. However, traumatic stress from direct patient care does not have to be from dealing with "blood and guts." Though seeing the type of trauma a human body will endure is traumatic, situational trauma can be equally devastating. It often has a greater impact on us due to the personal nature of it, which can cause us to be more drawn into the human side. In fact, there are times our emotions will surface when the physical trauma associated with the situation is not serious at all. In the previous example, my patients had relatively minor injuries. It was the loss of their father they had experienced, or were going to, that made the situation so difficult for me, since these kids were all the same ages as my own. There have been other times when just the situation alone was enough to affect me, even though the physical trauma the patient was dealing with was not that great.

Noodles

While working a travel assignment as a nurse in a small ER in the late part of my career, I had an experience that surprised me. I was at the tail end of my shift when our front registration person called to tell us there was a young man with burns at our front window. I walked out front to see the patient and found an eleven-year-old boy sitting at the desk with a very uncomfortable look on his face. As I could not see any apparent injury, I asked him what was up. He told me he was about to eat a bowl of Top Ramen when it spilled on his lap. I then noticed he was wearing sweatpants, and the front was wet.

I asked the woman who was with him if she was his mother. She told me he was one of her son's friends who was just at her house to play, and the mother was at work. The mother had been notified and was on her way to the ER, but since I know how severe scalding water can burn, and I had to assume his genitals may be involved, we brought him straight back to a room. In most cases, we would wait for parental permission. However, genital burns are considered major, so his situation was potentially "life or limb."

I walked him back to a treatment room and alerted the ER doctor to the situation. We agreed we needed to examine the burn to see if it warranted immediate treatment without waiting for a parent. I explained to this young boy as tenderly as I could that we were going to look at his burn and try to make him feel better and all that entailed. I helped him out of his clothes and into a gown. Once the doctor was in the room, I explained to the young man we needed to look at his "junk." Imagine this little boy in a room with strangers and no parents around. Now he is being asked to let us see and touch his penis and testicles. He was terrified but agreeable, and he lay back on the gurney.

On inspection, he had enormous blisters on both inner thighs. This was a pretty significant second-degree burn. However, there was no involvement of his genitals or danger to his reproductive organs. His eyes were wide as he lay there, letting us do what we needed to do. I explained everything to him. As gently as possible, we quickly applied a moist, sterile dressing and covered him up with a warm blanket. I told him I knew he must be very scared, but his parents would be so proud that he was being so brave. A tear began to stream down the side of his face. At that moment, my own eyes welled up, and my tears began to flow. It surprised me because this situation, dealing with a child before a parent arrives, is something I had encountered scores of times. However, this patient in this situation got to me openly. I smiled and told him, with tears streaming down my own face, it was okay to be scared and cry.

It surprised me how deeply affected I was and how emotional I became. I told him I would stay with him until his mother arrived. She finally got to the ER, and, as it often is with children, as soon as he saw her, he began to weep. She comforted him as I explained what happened and what his injury was, as well as the treatment we provided so far. I let her know we did not expose him while anyone was alone with him and only as briefly as was necessary. I then transferred care to the oncoming nurse and went home.

Over the years, I have seen colleagues affected differently during various situations. Often, there have been incidents I believed were pretty benign. I remember wondering why someone would be so deeply affected in such situations. I was drawn into the culture of, "This is the ER and not for the faint of heart." If you are easily affected by the things we deal with, perhaps you need to find another area of nursing to work in. I do not remember ever thinking people were weak or unreasonably emotional. I just thought it took an extra tough and calloused person to be able to effectively deal with the tragedies we deal with in the ER that other areas of healthcare do not. This is part of the toxic culture. Not realizing everyone is at a different place in their life and career when they encounter tragedies at work.

There is a pattern in these first three stories that will continue to play out in this book. Why it seems to be ignored or unnoticed is perplexing. So much time and energy is focused on the patient and family, as it should be. Yet it seems to be assumed those offering that attention are supposed to shake it off and get back to work. This is part of the toxic culture unique to my profession.

The first two examples were nearly thirty years apart. Yet the response to those providing the care was precisely the same. Nothing had changed in all those years. For me, I had been conditioned for decades to shake it off. Not only that, any mention of therapy was viewed by emergency services personnel as silly, and it was ridiculed by most of my colleagues. I am sure there were many who thought it might be a good idea. However, they kept that to themselves, for the most part. The culture of ignoring the psychological toll our experiences were having on us was deeply rooted. As I look back over the years, it seems nobody even considered the possibility of moral injury or traumatic stress being an issue. Even today, with more and more being written about it,

Silent Trauma: The side of healthcare we don't talk about

the culture of pretending moral injury does not occur dominates the emergency services industry.

BEARING WITNESS

"I have to realize it is their tragedy and not mine. When it is my tragedy, I will get emotionally drawn in, but I cannot do it when it is not my tragedy."

Brenda Little, RN

Page Hospital ER, Page, Arizona, 03/10/2022

There are times when the significant stress of the situation does not come from dealing directly with the patient; instead, the stress comes from dealing with those who are with the patient. Most of the time, these are the family members, but sometimes friends, of the patient. This is something that might be best described as a collateral stressor.

Ice Cream with Daddy

A young father was playing with his three-year-old daughter in their home. After a while, they decided to have ice cream cones together. About halfway through their ice cream, the young girl began to cry, holding her head. She complained of a headache. The father took the ice cream and offered her a drink of room-temperature water. This did not stop the child from crying. The parents both assumed the child had a "brain freeze" headache from the cold ice cream.

The father took the child to the bathroom and placed her in a warm tub to try and soothe her. Most parents might wonder what was happening; however, this was no ordinary parent. The father was an experienced emergency medicine physician. As he tried to console his child, he began to notice she was becoming lethargic. He also noticed one of her pupils was slightly larger than the other one. This is a very ominous sign. He had his wife call 911.

They were rushed to the emergency room where I was working. I was not the assigned nurse; rather, I was the team leader of the POD this patient was brought to. The patient was now almost completely unresponsive, and her breathing was abnormal. She was quickly intubated, placed on a ventilator, and taken for a CT scan of her brain. The news was not good. The little girl had suffered a spontaneous bleed in her brain. Her head was filling with blood, and the pressure was getting dangerously high. This is something we see often, but just not in children without a traumatic injury. What happens is that a blood vessel in the brain develops a small bubble, called an aneurysm, that grows until it pops. Two very significant things will happen. The area of the brain that was being fed oxygenated blood is now starved because the blood is not getting there. Also, the blood that is leaking out of the popped bubble is leaking into the surrounding tissue of the brain. Since the brain is enclosed in the skull, there is no visible swelling. Instead, there is just an ever-increasing pressure inside the skull that squeezes the entire brain from inside.

Because there are no outward signs of injury, it can be difficult for the family to understand the gravity of what is happening inside the body. It is sometimes counterintuitive to see someone who looks completely normal and yet is so gravely ill. This child looked very peaceful as she lay there on the ventilator. Seeing this perfect little angel lying there was difficult for everyone involved. However, I was not the patient's nurse.

My job was to help make certain the primary nurse had all the resources he needed to be able to do his job. My job, in part, was also to address the parents' needs with the social worker, who took the lead with the family. They were both sitting next to the bed, watching everything in complete silence. We were speaking to the father in hospital lingo because he was one of us and understood. The mother sat and just stared at her baby while holding her hand. I wondered why the father was not explaining everything to the mother. Perhaps he did not want her to know how ominous the situation was. The look of despair on the face of the parents was haunting. The father looked on, helpless to save his child, in spite of all his years of medical training.

We did not have the child for an extremely long period of time. She needed immediate surgery on her brain to relieve the pressure and try to save her young life. As a father and grandfather, I could not help but empathize with these parents. I had a grandchild who was the same age. I could not imagine what was going through their minds. It was emotionally draining.

When things like this happen, there is a different air in the department. Even with scores of other patients and family members coming in and out of the ER, there is a noticeable quiet among all the staff. News traveled fast about what was going on with this patient. Staff in the entire department could feel the tension and darkness that seemed to encompass the room this little family was in. We had a social worker there to stay with the parents. We made sure they had water or coffee or a warm blanket to make them comfortable. Our staff was continuously checking on them to make sure they had everything they needed. The social worker made phone calls to other family members for them and was by their side most of the time, accompanying the parents out of the ER when the child went to surgery. The rest of us? We went back to work.

No debriefing.
No offer of assistance.

Dealing with family members is often more traumatic for the staff than taking care of the patient. While seeing someone agonize in pain is difficult, we can give them medications to ease their suffering. Physical suffering, in most cases, has a treatment. Even if the patient does not survive, they are at peace. However, what do you do for someone whose suffering is emotional? The irony is we all discuss this in the ER. We talk about how tragic this is for the family. We recognize the long road to emotional recovery they will have after dealing with such a traumatic event. Yet we completely skip over the fact we have experienced it as well. We are obviously not personally involved like family and friends are. I would never make that comparison. However, we have experienced someone else's trauma. And we do it over and over and over again.

WHEN THE REASSURANCE FAILS

There are times when dealing with family members includes reassuring them and letting them know everything will be all right. I have been asked countless times, "How bad is this?" or "Is he going to be okay?" or "I am not sure what to do. What would you do if it were your own mother?" Trying to reassure patients and family members is something often overlooked as a stressor.

When someone experiences a laceration or broken bone or a myriad of other relatively minor injuries or illnesses, it is pretty easy to reassure them, knowing the outcome is almost guaranteed. However, when the circumstances are not so cut-and-dry, it can be more difficult. If we tell them we do not know, we may sound like we are not very experienced. On the other hand, we do not want to give false hope or create fear that may sway their treatment decision. If we persuade them to do one thing or the other, and they choose an option they regret, we may feel responsible for what happened.

Still, it is our job to help patients and family members make informed decisions. At times, this means encouraging them to go home after we have treated them, but many people feel more comfortable when they are with us in case they need help. This most often happens out of fear they will have a problem when nobody is around to help. In these cases, emergency workers must be confident in the service that was rendered and gently push the patient out the door to be discharged. We must reassure the patient and their family that everything is as good as it can be, and it is safe for them to go home. Sometimes, however, this can backfire in a big way.

The Radio Call

I worked with a particular nurse in the ER named Sande Burke. On this day, we started work at 6 a.m. Most ERs are at their lowest census at this time of morning. Though one of the busiest in California, on this day, our ER was pretty empty. There was a woman who had been in the ER all night with her eighteen-month-old little boy. He came in with asthma-type symptoms and had several breathing treatments through the night and some oral steroids. The night doctor and respiratory therapist said the child was ready for discharge, but the mother was resisting.

The newly arrived day shift doctor and respiratory therapist examined the boy, and said he looked great. His lungs were perfectly clear, and he was playfully and appropriately responding to his mother. Sande said he would go in and try to get them discharged. He was a very experienced nurse whom I admired and looked to for guidance. He had mentored me when I was new to the emergency department. He had previously been a respiratory therapist for many years before becoming a nurse. He was soft-spoken, with a very compassionate demeanor, and he had an innate ability to get people to trust him.

Sande went in and spoke with the mother. He also examined the boy and listened to his lung sounds. Perfectly clear! He told the mother it was time to take her son home. The mother resisted and said, "I know you are all saying he is fine, but there is just something that is not right with him." Sande persisted and assured the mother the child was ready to go. He told her she could come back if the slightest symptom reappeared. Reluctantly, the mother acquiesced and signed the discharge paperwork.

When Sande came out of the room, he was quite impressed with himself for being able to convince the mother to take the boy home, as I would have been. He shared with me how great the boy looked and that he had been appropriately and effectively treated in the night.

Several hours later, the familiar alarm of the paramedic radio sounded. In our county, there were specially trained nurses who would answer the radio and give the paramedics direction, if needed, on the treatment of their patients. Sande and I both entered the radio room, but he got to the radio first. He picked up the radio and answered it. The response was one that always stops you in your tracks: "Base, this is Squad 33 with a pediatric full arrest." Sande did not skip a beat and responded, "33, go ahead with your full arrest." The paramedic then said, "We have an eighteen-month-old boy who was discharged from your ER this morning after being there all night with a respiratory issue." Sande was visibly and understandably upset. He said to me, "Brian, there is no way I can be here when this mother gets here. Can you finish this call?" I picked up the radio and finished directing the call.

After speaking with the medics and giving them the orders they were requesting, I went out to let the team know what was coming. We set up the room to receive them when they arrived. Sande had gone to the manager's office to let her know the situation and remained there. I must add, there is nothing Sande did wrong. I would have done the same thing and encouraged this mother to take her child home.

When the child arrived, we had a team of the best people I have ever worked with tending to him. We worked tirelessly, attempting to resuscitate this sweet little boy. We did everything humanly possible to revive him. After we worked on the child for a very, very long time, the physician asked the question none of us want to hear, especially when the patient is a child: "Can anyone think of anything we have not done or could try?" With no reply from the team, he asked the final, more ominous question: "Does anyone have any objection to calling this?" (This means stopping our efforts.) With no objections, the decision was made by the team to suspend any further efforts.

I say the team because even though it is, ultimately, the responsibility of the physician to pronounce a patient dead, every doctor includes the team in the decision. This is a wise approach, since there could be something not done, and resuscitation is always a team effort. Perhaps it also allows the physician to feel less individually responsible and prevents them from wondering if they tried everything. This is a decision you must get right. The official time of death of this little boy was announced by the doctor.

In a room that had been bustling with activity and noise, you could now hear a pin drop. This is one of the most difficult decisions an emergency worker will ever be a part of. I always find myself staring at the body and wondering what this person might have become. It is a sobering moment for all involved.

The ER doctor asked me to go to the family room with him to inform the mother. We had our social worker in the room with them. As we entered the room, we saw the mother sitting on the floor. Her head was in the lap of her sister, who was sitting on the couch. The ER doctor and I did not have to say a word. It was all over our faces. The mother screamed, "NO!" and began to sob. Her sister looked at me with tears streaming down her face. I was afraid to try and speak, for fear of crying. All I could do was shake my head. I usually offer my condolences. This time, I could not even get the words "I am so sorry for your loss" out of my mouth.

I have been asked on many occasions what the worst thing is I have ever experienced in my career. I am sure people expect to hear some crazy story of trauma and chaos. However, the answer I give is always the same. That is, there is nothing more tragic or more heart-wrenching in this world than listening to the sobs of a mother who has just lost her child. The social worker stayed with the mother and her sister. Sande had the opportunity to go home if he wanted. I don't remember if he did. The rest of us went back to work.

No debriefing.
No offer of assistance.

FROM QUIET TO CHAOS TO QUIET AGAIN

The job of caring for other human beings can be a stressful one in the best of circumstances. Especially in emergency services, the stress level is high. Emergency caregivers are nearly always on edge—always needing to be prepared for the "what if" situation—even if it is subtle.

In the book *Emergency!* by Dr. Mark Brown (1997), he talks about "the doors," which refers to the doors of the ER. Mark shares stories from colleagues about the various things that will present at "the doors." Those of us on the inside of those doors have inherent anticipation of what might be on the other side when they open. This is very unique to the ER. As pointed out in Mark's book, and in this one, we can have a day of minor illnesses and injuries and, without notice, be presented with a critical patient who is dropped off. Though this can be an exciting part of emergency services, it also brings a unique kind of stress. Depending on how busy the ER is, it can sometimes feel like you are on edge, waiting for the shoe to drop. Sometimes you get a heads up, and sometimes it completely surprises you.

Family Feud

While doing my prerequisite studies for nursing school, I was working as a tech in an emergency room. We were a small ER with eight beds. There was another hospital in town, a large trauma center. I remember being frustrated that EMS did not bring trauma and other serious patients to us. As I matured in my career, I look back and realize that was wise. We were ill-equipped to deal with serious trauma patients. We had a very broad range of services for a small hospital. Even with just a twelve-bed ICU, our hospital performed open-heart surgeries and cared for very sick patients. Still, trauma required a different level of care and services. So, we would get medically ill patients, but rarely any trauma. Our staffing in the ER was minimal, consisting of two nurses and one tech, who also served as the unit secretary. We were so slow, our doctors worked twenty-four-hour shifts.

One evening after dark, our registration alerted us to a woman who said there was someone in her car who needed help. I went outside with a wheelchair to investigate. There was a small alleyway beside the ER. It was completely dark at night with no lights, so it was difficult to see. However, there was a car parked with the passenger rear door open. Though it was dark, I saw a man who was lying face down, mostly on the floor, moaning and waving his arms over his head.

The interior of the car was dark maroon, and the man was black. In the extreme darkness, this made it difficult to see him. I asked him to sit up and talk to me. He ignored me and persisted in his moaning. I confess, I was early in my career but was already reaching a high level of cynicism. I just knew, in my mind, this man was overexaggerating whatever was bothering him and was just making my job more difficult.

I became stern with him and told him to sit up, or I would not be able to help. I asked the woman what was wrong with him, and she said he had been in a fight: "I think his sister might have stabbed him with a knife." This got my attention. I was outside alone. I asked her to go inside and tell them I needed someone else to come out and help me, and to bring a gurney. I continued to try and get the man to turn over. I realized his moans seemed to be more agony than drama.

A nurse came outside with a gurney and asked me what was wrong. I told her I was not sure, but this man might be suffering from a stab wound. I reached down and grabbed him under both of his arms. As I pulled him toward me, he was slipping from my grasp. He seemed very sweaty, and it was hard to keep hold of him. He was not helping me at all. I pulled him toward me and against my legs. I then got a better grip on him and pulled him out. I bent my knees and put them under his chest to help me leverage him up to the gurney. The nurse I was with looked at me and gasped. We wore white pants back then. I looked down, and my pants were completely red. This man was not sweating; he was bleeding very badly.

We quickly took him into the ER. His blood pressure was extremely low, and his heart was racing. He and I were completely covered in his blood. Soon after, he lost a pulse, and we began CPR. Remember, we had two nurses, one doctor, and me. There was no trauma team to activate. We called for help, and a respiratory therapist arrived. Miraculously, one of our cardiovascular (CV) surgeons was in the hospital and walked into the ER. He just happened to be passing through to get to the parking lot so he could go home. He was wearing a T-shirt, shorts, and flip-flops. He asked if he could help, and we were all happy to let him jump in.

We saw a small stab wound in the patient's upper-left chest. The ER doctor told the surgeon we needed to open the chest immediately. The surgeon donned gloves and was presented with the thoracotomy tray, which is a tray with sterile instruments needed to emergently open a chest. Normally, he had a surgical tech who knew what all the instruments in the kit were and would pass them to him. This time, he only had me, an ER tech who had no idea what was in the tray. However, with him pointing to things, I was able to get him what he needed.

The CV surgeon had the chest open in seconds. He quickly discovered a small stab wound in the left atrium of the heart. He cut off a small piece of the pericardium, the membrane surrounding the heart, and sutured it over the hole. He then had me put a finger on top of the patch and massage the heart. My adrenaline was rushing through me.

This was not the first time I had seen a chest opened in the ER. However, this time, I had my hands inside the chest and was squeezing this man's heart as the surgeon directed me, manually pumping blood through a human body. I was consumed with the thought that I had this man's life in my hands, literally. My heart was racing, and I remember sweating.

The surgeon obtained small defibrillation paddles to shock the heart directly. In a matter of minutes, the heart was beating on its own. However, there was so much blood loss, the beating of his heart did not last long. After a long time of resuscitation efforts, the patient was ultimately pronounced dead. In just a few seconds, we went from complete, controlled chaos with lots of activity to virtual silence. I was standing there, resting my hands inside this man's chest cavity. Blood was up my arms, past the gloves I was wearing. I stared into this open chest, looking at the heart, aorta, and left lung. I remember staring at this young man's face and wondering what had transpired between his sister and him. I went from feeling superhuman in the middle of this crisis to completely helpless.

Though I remain skeptical when I hear someone's story, this incident taught me not to be dismissive. As the Russian saying, made popular by Ronald Reagan, goes . . . I have adopted the mantra of "Trust but verify."

The room was cleaned, the coroner took the body, and we went back to sitting around not doing much. Just like that, the atmosphere had reverted to what it was before this completely chaotic event hit our little ER. We all went back to work.

No debriefing.
No offer of assistance.

RECOGNIZING THE EMOTIONAL IMPACT
OF WHAT WE DO

Where is the line between professionalism in the face of crisis and personalizing what we encounter? We are human beings. We are wired for compassion and sorrow in the face of tragedy. We also have an amazing, innate ability to keep it together in chaotic situations so we might perform the tasks necessary for survival. Sometimes we must do all of this at the same time. Especially in the ER, where we never get patients one at a time. We do not encounter a situation and then, even occasionally, have the opportunity of returning to quarters or base of operations, and get a short break before the next tragedy.

I am not diminishing the impact of traumatic stress on first responders or other departments in the hospital. They deal with the same tragedies we do in the emergency room. There is, however, a distinct difference in the situations faced by those who work in emergency rooms. We can never go out of service. We can never stop accepting patients if all our beds are full. We can never close to patients because we are short-staffed. We care for a multitude of patients with widely varying levels of need continuously. The doors can never close!

Our ability as humans to compartmentalize tragedy and keep pressing forward is not unique to emergency services workers. Look at the pioneers in the early days of the United States. A study was done of early Mormon pioneers (Bashore & Tolley, 1994). Many kept good journals, so details of their travels are readily available. Approximately 4% of those traveling across the country died. Men, women, and children were among those who perished, but the remaining fathers, mothers, and siblings all had to press forward and continue the journey. Since the beginning of time, people have dealt with tragedy and pushed through it.

Those in emergency services are not new to this phenomenon. However, the daily exposure to human tragedy and situations of despair takes its toll on those who experience it. I am not diminishing the impact on anyone who works in healthcare or serves in combat or excluding them from anything of what I am speaking of. I am simply focused on what I have an expertise in, and that is emergency services.

As previously stated, all are affected, in my opinion. Some of us believe we are not affected. I was always one of those. I had convinced myself I was not affected any longer by my work experiences. I had been doing this for so long and had experienced so many different types of tragedies that I was certain I was solid and was completely unaffected by anything I experienced. I knew how to deal with it, and there was no pent-up trauma waiting to burst out of me. I was convinced I had a special gift, like so many of my colleagues, of being able to handle anything I encountered without being affected in any way.

The Epiphany

Over the Christmas season in 2016, my wife and I were getting ready to fly to New Orleans. We were excited about the trip. We were living in Utah, but I still traveled to California to work. Before our trip to New Orleans, we had gone to California for me to work a couple of shifts, and then we would fly out of Los Angeles. The day we were to fly out, I needed to stop by work to check my email and approve my timecard so I could get paid, and my wife came with me. There were two nurses I needed to speak with. One was the nurse I was rooming with while working in

CA, and the other was the nurse who managed the schedule.

When we arrived at work, I asked where these nurses were and was told they were both in Room 21. This is one of our trauma and critical incident rooms. As we walked by the room, I could see there was a great commotion and several people around the bed. This is never a good sign in the ER. I have often told people who complain about the wait time that, "You never want to be first in the emergency room." I mentioned to my wife that they looked busy, so we would have to wait. We sat at the counter facing the room where there was a computer for me to use. There are huge observation windows between where we were sitting and the trauma bay because the ER was an academic facility, and the designers likely assumed there would be many people wanting to observe the traumas without being in the room. However, these windows had mini blinds on them, which were always closed, and so we could not see into the room.

At some point, I pulled the blinds back to look into the room and see when my colleagues might be finished so we could leave. As I looked into the room, I could see the team was performing CPR. The patient looked to be an elderly gentleman. I remember, once I realized what was going on in the room, saying aloud, "Oh, this won't last very long." My comment was based on the fact that CPR on the elderly often does not have a good outcome. It was also my hope, I am ashamed to say, that it would not last long, and I could speak with these two nurses so we would be able to get out of there sooner rather than later.

I went back to my email and, at some point, said something to my wife. When she did not respond to me, I looked over at her. She was sitting there with tears streaming down her face. I asked her what was wrong. She just looked at me and said, "You guys do this every day!" At first, I was not sure what she was talking about. I said something like, "We do what every day?" She just shook her head and did not say much more about it. However, when we were at the airport, waiting for our flight, she made a social media post. Here is the exact text of her post:

We live and we learn; sometimes a little at a time and sometimes one big eye-opening lesson all at once. I hear about days in the crazy CA ER all the time, and I honestly have had a decent amount of sympathy for the talent, skill, tolerance, compassion, AND callous it must take to effectively work there for years. But I just had an experience that gave me much more insight.

As I sat at a computer in the ER waiting for Brian to check his email, etc. . . . I got a glimpse of a man in the next room having CPR administered. I witnessed a family member nervously pacing outside another room, waiting for a doctor to explain the gravity of their loved one's situation. I hear of two patients with gunshot wounds being cared for . . . while another woman with far less serious issues yells at a nurse to get her a ginger ale as if she's at the Ritz Carlton, basing her tip on good service and completely oblivious to the devastation going on.

I watch nurses and doctors go from one enormous train wreck of a situation to another and joke with each other or exchange small talk in between. I recall stories of my husband and others like him dealing with things like having to tell parents about a child dying unexpectedly, while someone in the next room is furious because they've waited 2 hours to be seen for a rash.

My husband LOVES people. He takes the time to learn about the lives and history of his patients, which makes it even harder to deal with and explain their sometimes awful prognosis. My eyes filled up with tears. One half hour as a bystander in the midst of lives changing and ending around me, and my heart broke. Although I see the other side . . . the soft-hearted, loving guy, sometimes Brian can seem abrasive or less than sympathetic. Aha moment: This is partially why he is SO good at what he does. One with such a romantic heart cannot live this daily without building up some callous, sarcasm, humor, and a sense of; assess the facts, do the tasks well and quickly, and then "suck it up and move on!" and "Oh, I'm super sorry you had to wait for your damn ginger ale while I got someone else's heart beating and stopped another's profuse bleeding!"

Sometimes, things we find undesirable in others are in some way the very things they were put here on earth to do. I couldn't do what he and so many he works with do. I have a deeper appreciation for him, for them, and for others whose talents or life experiences I have not understood or appreciated in the past.

Wow! Sitting in the airport, I read that and suddenly realized there were many things about my job that generate a significant emotional response in a human being. My wife was not a wimp. She had many trials in life that had hardened her resolve and made her solid in the face of adversity. But this really affected her. For the first time, I began to ask myself why I was not affected by all of this. Or was I? As I read her post, my eyes welled with tears. Tears for my wife, who I callously exposed to this without any thought of how she may be affected. Tears for my colleagues, who were the ones she watched and spoke of. And tears for myself for suddenly, after three decades, realizing how I *should* be feeling.

The incident in the ER with my wife and her subsequent social media assessment really got me thinking about everything my coworkers and I have experienced over the years. What had I actually seen, and why was I seemingly not affected by it any longer, if ever?

During this same trip, we encountered a situation that sparked another social media discussion. It had to do with people who, in my opinion, abuse the claim of "stress" to gain access to priorities for travel. Rather ironic, considering the subject of this book. I made a snarky post about people who abuse the claim of "service animal."

In my post, I specifically mention I was not talking about actual trained service animals. In the discussion, I was being attacked for not understanding what stress really was. I was lectured by many people who would relate stories of a spouse or friend or family member who served in combat. They would tell me how hard these people had it and how difficult it was for them every day. I revere our soldiers and never suggested they did not suffer from stress. These were not the people I was referring to who were abusing the system, and I had made that very clear in my post. However, the barrage of comments rebuking me seemed endless.

One particular comment sent me over the edge. It suggested I had no idea what it is like to live with someone who has experienced real stress and that I should "live a day in their shoes" so I would know what traumatic stress is really like. This comment, for some reason, sparked something in me, and I was fuming. I thought, "How dare this person assume I do not know what stress is?" I was angry and took offense, so I wrote an instant reply. I did not have to pause to collect my thoughts. Without thinking, I just started typing and then sent my message without reading it. My reply, in part, was:

[Okay], time to respond to all the posts[. . . .] I work in healthcare. All the anecdotal stories here are not increasing my exposure to people with real issues, nor are they dissuading me from anything previously stated. Now, for those of you who think I need to spend a day in your shoes, let me enlighten you. From the age of seventeen, I have personally watched literally, hundreds of people die. From infants who were abused to the elderly who passed peacefully. I have seen death and injury from poisoning, gunshots, hangings, stabbings, burns, explosions, aircraft crashes, drownings, diseases, starvation, beatings, falls, vehicle accidents, strangling, torture, and allergic reactions. I have seen brains, bones, guts, fingers, toes, eyeballs, ears, arms, legs, and heads separated from where they belong. I have had many of the aforementioned anatomical parts on me. Of course, I have seen more blood than any of you will ever realize. I have listened to screams, moans, and cries! I have had people begging me to make the pain stop and heard, "Please help me," infinitely more than I have ever heard, "Thank you." I have had family members

beg me to do more and tell me why their loved one just has to be saved because they are so important to so many people. I have watched hundreds of parents anguish over the loss of their child, and in many cases was the one who told them of the passing. I have heard the worst sound ever more times than I can recount; mothers quietly sobbing at the loss of their beautiful child. I have tried to comfort countless people who have lost someone while trying to fight back my own tears and sometimes crying with them. I have seen every bit of trauma that can happen to a human body and more than most people commenting here can even begin to imagine. I have walked out of rooms where people are fighting for their lives with blood all over the walls, floor, and some of the staff, and into a room to tend to a small child with a tummy ache, and I am expected to slap on a happy face and not let what I just witnessed 60 seconds ago show to my new patient. I stood on a hill and watched the coroner remove charred pieces of the bodies of three of my friends from the medical helicopter they were flying in when it crashed and burned. All these things I have personally experienced and not just heard about from a loved one or friend. I have personally experienced things beyond what nearly every person commenting on this thread can even imagine, so please do not lecture me on traumatic stress! I don't need to "come spend a day in your world"! My reality has given me a far clearer picture about what I am talking, than the well-intentioned examples cited by those commenting here.

After I sent that message, I was still fuming. My wife calmed me down, and we went to sleep. However, when I woke up the next morning, I went back and reread what I had posted. I had typed it so fast, I honestly did not remember what I wrote. As I read it, I had this sick feeling in my stomach. I actually *had* experienced everything I typed in my post. Nothing was an exaggeration or embellishment. It was overwhelming, and I began to cry. So much so that I could hardly read through the tears. My career seemed to have flown by, and yet I had actually experienced everything I was reading and more. I also realized something I had not considered before. Perhaps I **was** affected by my experiences.

HEALTHCARE ADMINISTRATION'S APPROACH TO CRITICAL EVENTS

During the writing of this book, I had an experience which highlights my message very well. While there are a couple of good examples of the staff looking out for each other, this incident illustrates how the organization failed to address the serious emotional toll on the staff, even after it was brought to the senior leadership's attention. I want to stress again, this is not meant to paint the organization in a bad light. My research for this book tells me this example is more "the rule" in my industry, rather than "the exception."

The Debriefing that Never Came

I was working in the ER as a primary nurse in one of our four trauma assignments. This meant I was assigned four beds—two trauma and two general. I was notified by the charge nurse a "Level 1" trauma was being activated and would be coming to one of my rooms. Level 1 meant it was the most serious of traumas. While preparing to receive the patient, I was given a preliminary report by Sheila Anulao, the nurse who received the radio call. A sixty-year-old female with a self-inflicted gunshot wound to the head, with brain matter showing. I immediately questioned the likelihood of the patient making it to us alive. Sheila told me she had questioned the paramedic crew about that same thing over the radio. She asked them about the patient's status, considering the grave initial report. She tried to sway them toward pronouncing death in the field, since the patient met the criteria for consideration. She said the paramedics were pretty dismissive of this advice. They informed her the patient had a strong pulse and good blood pressure, so they would be transporting the patient.

The discussion in the room among the trauma team was mostly about how quickly this would likely be over once the patient arrived. However, we were prepared for a full-court press and to give the patient the best care we could. In our trauma activations, the primary nurse was the scribe, being responsible for all documentation and making sure the information flowed from the lead trauma surgeon to the team and back. The primary nurse would not participate in the initial hands-on care. This was the responsibility of at least two additional nurses and several ER technicians, along with the trauma physicians and other ancillary team members (respiratory, lab, X-ray, CT, pharmacy, social services, admitting, surgery team, EMS crews, blood bank). Ideally, there was an initial "swarming" of the patient: addressing the airway, getting intravenous access, lab draws, administering blood products, X-rays, identification of family, registration, etc. As tasks were completed, team members who were no longer needed would fall out and go back to their other assignments in the ER. Eventually, the primary nurse is left as the primary caregiver, either alone or with whatever resources are required to adequately care for the patient.

Once the team was assembled, we were advised the ambulance had arrived and would be in momentarily with the patient. Sheila, the nurse who took the radio call, was waiting at the trauma room entrance for the patient and would be one of the nurses initially completing bedside tasks. As the patient was coming down the hall, Sheila turned to me with a horrified look and said, "Oh my gosh, this is not a sixty-year-old."

At that moment, the patient appeared in the doorway with EMS. It was just a kid! Though much was happening, the room became quiet so we could all hear the report from the paramedics. "This is a sixteen-year-old female from home with a self-inflicted gunshot wound to the side of the head. There was grey [brain] matter at the scene. Her eighteen-year-old brother was in the house and heard the shot. He ran to his room and immediately called 911. She has strong central and peripheral pulses and good blood pressure." They continued with reporting the care they had provided thus far. They added there was someone on FaceTime, video chatting with the patient when she shot herself. They told us they could hear someone screaming and crying when they entered the room and found her phone with a boy on the other end, still connected. Then they said, "Her father is a local fire captain and her mother is a paramedic." At some point, Sheila came to me and told me how sick she felt for not being more understanding of the paramedics, on the radio, wanting to bring the patient in. She told me how shocked she was to see a young teen, the same age as her son, and not a grown woman. She was clearly very upset.

Though none of us knew this young woman or her family, it instantly becomes more real when you realize the patient or their family is in our line of work, either medical or otherwise. In our traumas, we have social workers who are amazing. During the chaos of the medical attention, they weave in between us to get patient information as quickly as possible so they can address the emotional needs of the patients and their family members. Everyone knew this was going to be different because the patient's parents were members of a local fire department. Our social workers are on the front line of dealing with families, and this case was going to be exceptionally emotional.

Once we completed our initial stabilization of the patient, we took her to the CT scanner. This is quite an ordeal in these cases. The patient has multiple IV lines with medication, fluids, and blood infusing. She is also intubated and on a ventilator. To get her to CT requires portable monitors, IV pumps, a transport ventilator, at least one RN, a respiratory therapist, at least one ER tech, and all the supplies and emergency medication necessary to intervene should the patient become more unstable and go into cardiac arrest.

The primary ER tech assigned to me was Tyler Rochford. He was an experienced tech who was also a new paramedic awaiting a start date with one of our local fire departments. He was with me from the initial receiving of this patient until we ultimately delivered her to the ICU. The team took the patient to CT and back without incident. The report, though not surprising, was grave. The bullet had passed from one side of the head to the other and out. The injury to the brain was devastating and catastrophic. In the words of the attending trauma surgeon: it was "an unsurvivable injury."

Once back from the CT scanner, the social worker informed me the father was in the quiet room and would like to come see the patient. She also informed me there were unique family dynamics at play. The parents were no longer married. Mom was remarried, and the patient's parents had a volatile relationship. Apparently, the patient's parents had not been in the same room together for a very long time. There were many fire department brass in the hospital to support the parents and to help "keep the peace," if needed. Plans were underway to facilitate another quiet room to keep the parents separated. The fire department had sent one of their helicopters to get the mother, who was in a neighboring city.

The primary trauma surgeon went with the social worker to speak with the father. Upon returning, he told me the father really wanted to come in, and I wanted him to come in. As a father, I would want to be by my child's side in this circumstance. I asked the surgeon what he had told the father. He said the family was told the injury was not survivable. I asked him if he had told the family about how the patient appeared at the moment. He had not. I told the social worker I would like to go speak with the family before they came into the room.

I have spoken with many family members. It is something I do not necessarily mind doing. Over the years, I believe I have developed the ability to modify my approach based on the parties involved and their respective situations. However, it is something I do with reverence for those involved.

As I entered the quiet room with the social worker, there were four people present. The patient's father and sister were there, as well as the ER manager and chief nursing officer. Initially, I was a bit surprised to find them in the room. It was very unusual to see them directly involved in this type of thing. However, due to the circumstances, this was a high-profile public relations incident, so the leadership of the hospital was notified. There was also an enormous fire department presence. Not rank-and-file firefighters, but high-ranking brass.

I immediately approached the father, who stood up. I introduced myself and told the father and sister I was the primary nurse caring for their family member. The patient's sister was there with blood on her clothing and both hands. She was at her sister's side first and had still refused to wash her hands. Knowing the father is a fire captain and having encountered similar family members before, I knew he would be initially in "fireman mode" rather than "dad mode." I addressed him and said, "Listen, I know you are in the biz, but this is your kid, and I need you to understand what she looks like right now." He responded, "I know. I saw her on the gurney being taken somewhere earlier." I told him, even in that short amount of time, his daughter's appearance had changed rather dramatically. I described the ventilator and wires and tubes. I explained that with a devastating injury like this, the brain swells significantly. I shared how her head was rather large, and her eyes were severely swollen and purple. I said, "I know you have seen many terrible things in your career. However, when it is a close family member, it changes things. No matter how prepared you think you are for what you are about to see, it will likely take your breath away when you first enter the room." With that, the father said he needed to use the restroom before seeing his daughter.

I went back to the patient and left the family with the social worker. A short time later, the father and the sister entered the room with the social worker. Nothing I write could adequately describe the profound sorrow on the faces of these good people when they entered the room. I, and my tech Tyler, stepped back across the room to give them as much privacy as the circumstances would allow. They both looked at this young girl. The sister wept aloud as she apologized to her sister for not being there to look after her. She told her how wonderful and kind and generous she was. She told her how loved she was and how many people she had touched in her life. The father tried to keep a stiff upper lip. He quietly wept while holding his daughter's hand. It was profoundly emotional. I looked at Tyler, and his eyes welled up, on the verge of overflowing. I asked him if he was okay. He said, "This is terrible. I have never experienced anything like this before."

After some time, the father and sister thanked us and left the room. Almost immediately, the social worker told me the mother was here. She had told the mother I would want to speak with her before she came in to see the patient. She said the mother refused and was outside the room, insisting on coming in right now. There was no way I was going to try to delay this mom wanting to come in, and so I asked the social worker to let her come in. The mother came in, accompanied by the patient's sister. As previously stated, I believe there is nothing more tragic than the sobs of a mother who is grieving the loss of her child. This mother went to her daughter and took her hand. She touched her face and begged her to wake up. She knew the extent of her injury. She had been told it was a fatal wound. As a paramedic, she knew in her heart what the outcome would be. However, she was not a medic on this day. She was a mother. This was her daughter. Reason and logic are never at play in these situations, even for the most seasoned of emergency service workers, when the patient is your family member. This mother wanted her daughter to wake up and look at her. She fell to her knees next to the bed and wept. Her daughter comforted her. All Tyler and I could do was watch and try to take it all in. Tears streamed down my own cheeks as I stood there watching this mother's heart completely shatter, wishing I could do something to ease her pain. Part of me also prayed, silently, that I would never find myself in her situation, grieving over a child.

After some time, the social worker came into the room and gestured toward me. She said the father was outside and would like to come back in. I relayed this request to the patient's mother. She looked up at me and said, "Yes, that would be fine." A moment later, the social worker came back in with the father. There were also four high-ranking firefighters and the ER manager there to "keep the peace" with the parents. This seemed like quite an intrusion. They all stood at the foot of the bed, just staring at the patient and her family. The father approached the foot of the bed and knelt down. This broken little family wept together. After a few minutes, the patient's sister looked up at the firefighters and my manager and said, "Can everyone who does not need to be in here leave the room, please? We would like to have some privacy." With that, the firefighters and ER manager exited the trauma room. Tyler and I sank back as far as we could into the corner to be as invisible as possible. I am not going to share the conversation this family had. They discussed many things, including how this could possibly happen. I watched in awe as the patient's sister, a devastated eighteen-year-old, helped facilitate productive communication between her parents.

After a while, the father and sister left the room. The mother would not leave her daughter's side. During this entire encounter, we were supporting the patient's blood pressure with medication. As in all situations like this, even when death is certain, we know there is a possibility of saving many other lives through the miraculous gift of organ donation. Until a patient has been declared brain-dead, though, it is not okay to discuss donation with the family.

Eventually, we received a room assignment and gathered the team to transport the patient upstairs to the ICU. The mother, who had not stopped holding the patient's hand, insisted on doing so during the transport. Except for narrow passages where she could not physically be beside the gurney, she never let her go. Upon arrival at the ICU, I pleaded with the mother to please wait outside the room until we moved her over. I explained to her about the large number of staff it would require to carefully move her over, that we could not do it while she held her hand, and that she would only be a few steps away from her should her condition change. Seeing all the people in the room, she acquiesced and agreed to wait outside the room.

Just as we moved the patient over, while all the support staff were still in the room, I noticed the mother step into the room. She was standing by the door and motioned to me. When I walked over, she asked, "Brian, I noticed there are sutures on the side of my daughter's head. Was her skull blown apart? Did they have to piece her head back together?" Now, I am one who is never at a loss for words. But I just stood there, face-to-face with this mother, and tried to process what she just asked me. After a few seconds, I motioned toward the hall and asked her to join me outside the room. This was partly a stall to collect my thoughts. I also did not want to have this discussion in the room with other people around. Once we were in the hall, I turned to face her. I placed my hands on her arms and said, "Listen, I understand you are in the biz and have seen some horrific things in your career. But this is not the time to be a medic. That is your daughter lying in there. You do not want those kinds of details, and I do not want to share them with you. Please, I beg of you, don't ask me to tell you those details." She paused briefly and then put her head on my chest and began to cry. She said, "You are right. I don't want to know. I don't know why I even asked you that." I assured her it was okay, that she was not on trial, being judged. She had just been hit with a devastating, life-changing event that she was just beginning to process. She tried to regain her composure and then went back into the room.

As I began to head back to the ER, I saw the sister standing in the hallway. I felt compelled to talk with her. I asked her if I could speak with her for a minute, and we stepped around the corner. I asked her how she was doing. I commended her for being so stoic in such a traumatic situation, as well as for being so mature in the face of her parents coming together and asking everyone to leave the room. I then asked her what she thought the outcome was going to be for her sister. She said, "Well, I know she is going to die." Hearing her say this choked me up a bit, but it confirmed her understanding of the situation.

I then went against policy and told her I was going to discuss something I was not supposed to. I asked her if she had ever heard of people donating organs. She told me she had and was already wondering if that would be a possibility with her sister. I explained to her a little about the process and told her, though we were not supposed to approach the family yet, she could ask to speak with the representatives from One Legacy, the organization that coordinates the donation process. I explained how many lives could be saved by the process and how her family might be able to help others through her sister's tragedy. She explained to me how much her sister loved to help other people and how that is exactly what she would want. She asked me what she should do, and I gave her some direction about whom to speak with. I then left her so I could return to the ER.

Immediately upon returning to the ER, the resource nurse who had been taking care of my other assigned beds for the last six hours while I was with my trauma patient approached me and asked if I was ready for a report on the other patients in my assignment. You see, this is the culture—to "get back to work." Before I could answer, the nurse who was the team leader of my POD, Vandy, intervened and said, "Brian, why don't you walk away for a little while and clear your head. Go outside or find a quiet place to sit and come back when you are ready." This was not the policy of my department, nor was it initiated by anyone in a leadership role. It was an experienced, compassionate nurse who just happened to be assigned as team leader that day, rather than having her own assignment. I had not taken my lunch yet and decided this was a good time.

As I walked away to go to the cafeteria and get a bite, two other individuals approached me. Both were ER techs. The first was Edwin, who looked at me and, with a somber tone, said, "Man, bro, that was a pretty shitty deal." That was his way of saying, "I am with you and hope you are good." Right after that, a female tech, Ashley, walked up to me and put her hand on my shoulder. She looked me in the eyes and said, "Are you okay, Brian?" This brought tears to my eyes. Not because I was not okay. It was because these two colleagues, who had assignments in completely different PODS far from the trauma bay I spent the last six hours in, sought me out to make sure I was good. It made me so happy to know there are people who get it. They understand exactly what I am writing this book about. It also illustrated to me how catastrophic events in the ER affect the entire department. Our ER was set up in five separate PODS. Mini ERs, if you will. You really do not have any idea what is going on in the other areas. However, when big incidents happen, the word travels about what is going on and who the assigned staff are. After my lunch, I came back and went to work.

No debriefing.
No offer of assistance.
Just back to work.

At the end of my shift, I was in our break room with the rest of the day crew. We were all doing the clock watch, waiting to be able to clock out for the day. Tyler and I were sitting down, and virtually all the staff were standing around asking about our trauma and what had happened. Many were asking probing questions. They wanted details about the incident. These were not coworkers sitting around talking shop. They weren't looking for gruesome details. It was their way of debriefing through our experience. Being in the middle of writing this book, I was hyperaware of the need to debrief and detox from incidents like this. The discussion we were having made me keenly aware of how desperate my colleagues are for debriefings. It was a great experience for me and one I will not soon forget.

The next day, I was working and went up to the ICU to see how the family was doing. I found the mother at the bedside, holding a vigil. She welcomed me to sit with her. We talked for almost forty-five minutes. She told me all about her daughter—what a great kid she was. She recounted her past few years struggling with depression. She openly wondered what she might have done to contribute to her death and what more she could have done to prevent it. She shared that they had already declared her daughter brain-dead and were scheduling her for surgery in two more days to harvest her organs and tissues. It was still surreal for her, and she was still trying to wrap her head around the whole thing. She gave me her card and asked me to keep in touch.

As I walked away, I was still processing the entire event in my own mind, things I did and said. How I interacted with the family and my colleagues. I also wondered if anyone from my hospital would organize a debriefing for those involved and check to make sure everyone was okay. I was not very hopeful.

A few weeks later, I received a call from the chief nursing officer's executive assistant, informing me the CNO would like to meet with me. I had been trying to get a meeting with her for several months regarding other concerns I had about my department leadership. She was very busy, and I lived far away, so getting together was not easy. We scheduled a meeting for the following week when I would be at work. I was told I would have an hour of her time. I was super excited because I had been looking forward to speaking with her.

When the day for our meeting came, I reported off to another nurse who would cover me while I was gone. As I entered the CNO's office, she stood up and walked around her desk to greet me. There was a table in the front part of her office to my right, and I looked over and noticed a representative from human resources sitting at the table. I thought this was very odd since I had specifically requested a private meeting with the CNO, and she was aware of some of the things I meant to speak with her about. She shook my hand and invited me to sit down at the table. The first thing she said to me was, "I know I owe you a meeting, Brian, to discuss your concerns, and I promise you I will arrange that as soon as I have time. However, that is not why I asked to see you." My head was reeling as to why the CNO, four levels up my chain of command, wanted to speak with me in the presence of HR. I did not have to wait long to find out.

The CNO said, "Several weeks ago, there was a tragic event where a young woman shot herself in the head. I am sure you remember." I responded, "How could I not possibly remember?" She went on, "When you came into the quiet room to speak with the father, there were some people in the room who felt you were pretty harsh in dealing with him." I was shocked. She continued, "When you walked in, after greeting the father and introducing yourself, you said something like, 'I know you are in the biz, but this is your kid.' Some thought that was cold and uncaring." I asked, "Did the family express concerns about my approach to them?" She assured me it was not any of the family. I then became a little irritable. I responded to the CNO by simply stating, "Then I don't care!" This is clearly not the response she expected from me.

She went on to explain how the hospital is trying to foster an environment of caring communication, and "some" in the room felt I was less than sensitive to the family. I then said, "Well, the only people in the room were the father, the sister, my manager, the social worker, and you. So 'some people' narrows the field down to you, the social worker, and my manager." She acknowledged that she was taken aback a little by my approach to the father. I then explained to her why I took the approach I did. I explained how I suspected the father would be, at least partially, in firefighter mode. I wanted to speak shop to him, initially, to let him know I was speaking his language. I felt that if I used shoptalk, "I know you are in the biz," it would lower his defenses and open him up to what I was about to tell him. I explained to the CNO how the family had all thanked me for being direct and telling them the straight truth. I recounted my conversation with the mother in the ICU, when she was in medic mode, and I tried my best to redirect her back to mom mode. I knew the parents' work mode was their way of dealing with their emotions, as they had been conditioned to do in their profession. The CNO expressed relief at my explanation. She asked me if I understood how people could get the impression they did from what I said and how I said it. I acknowledged as much.

After clarifying my approach, the CNO said she was satisfied. Our meeting had, so far, only taken ten minutes. She asked if I would like to have the other discussion we had been planning since we had so much time left. I told her I would, but before excusing the HR representative, I wanted to share something else. I explained to her about this book. I shared with her my passion for trying to change the culture where employees do not feel safe expressing their emotions about critical incidents. I explained how I believed the culture is fostered by employees and organizations that do not address the issue head-on and do not routinely offer effective, critical incident stress debriefings. I told her how our hospital was going to make an appearance in my book. I then reminded her of the incident in question. Since she was in the quiet room with the family when I spoke with the father, she was aware of how emotional the event was for everyone. How emotionally affected she was without even experiencing the patient care and initial family visits to the bedside. She completely agreed about how devastating the event was for all involved.

I asked, "Do you want to know who the first person from this hospital in a leadership role was to come to me about this tragic event?" She said she would love to know. I then said, "It was you, just now, calling me into the office to tell me you thought I was rude to the father." There was a long, awkward silence while we just looked at each other.

I then shared with her the two techs who came to check on me and the impromptu debriefing we had at the end of the shift. I shared with her how productive that was for all involved. I told her how much it would mean for the staff to know their leadership was aware of this incident and was concerned for them. She then assured me there is a program in place in all the departments and how debriefings are conducted quite regularly in situations like this. It was as if she did not hear what I just told her. I responded, "Not in my department." I again told her she was the first person of leadership to talk to me, and it was a disciplinary meeting with HR. I told her, in the years I had worked in this facility, I had never experienced a person from leadership checking on the staff after an event like this. She was silent.

As I sit here writing this portion of my book, it has been thirteen months to the day of that incident. Even after bringing this to the attention of the CNO, there has still been no person from any level of leadership in my hospital to approach the staff. Nobody from management, employee engagement, social services, spiritual services, nobody! Everyone was expected to just go back to work.

No debriefing.

No offer of assistance.

I must say again, I am not pointing a finger at any particular organization or person. In fact, as I previously stated, organizations that get it right in this type of situation are, in my research, the exception and not the rule. For whatever reason, it seems the mental health of the staff in healthcare is just not a priority. In fact, the people side of most professions is likely not a priority.

I am not suggesting I have a corner on the market of having the perfect track record in these situations. When I was deep in my career, with many experiences in these situations, I encountered one of the most tragic situations I can remember.

Burned

I was working the greatest job in healthcare as a flight nurse. It was like not having a real job. I have never enjoyed doing something so much in my entire working life. Eventually, I became the chief flight nurse of my company's program. I had the best flight nurses, flight medics, pilots, and mechanics to work with. Our leadership team was amazing. Our helicopter pilots were the best, with strict requirements for hire. Our hiring requirements for nurses and medics were the steepest in the industry at that time. One had to be a seasoned and skilled professional to even apply for a job. The hiring process was grueling to ensure only the best of the best were on our flight teams. We responded to the sickest of the sick, and what we often did was not for the faint of heart. None were rookies, and all had their own experiences that built up their emotional callouses, helping them deal with the things they encountered every day. However, there is always something out there to rock even the most stoic of us.

One afternoon, a request came in for a helicopter to respond to an explosion at a manufacturing plant where road flares were made. A huge vat of hot chemicals exploded and covered two workers. Upon arrival, the two victims were in the back of separate ambulances. One had 70% second-degree and third-degree burns, and the other had greater than 90% third-degree burns. The second gentleman had burns covering his entire head, face, and neck, as well as most of the rest of his body. It is extremely rare for someone with burns this significant to survive. The problem is it can take several days for the mercy of death to come. Anyone who has burned their finger on the stove or had a bad sunburn knows how painful burns are. This man had major burns on his entire body. In the back of the ambulance, the scene was gruesome. The patient was on the gurney, and a paramedic was tending to him, making sure he did not lose his airway. They were giving him morphine through a device drilled into his bone because they could not find any veins through the charred flesh. The smell was atrocious. Everyone, including the man with the burns, knew the outcome was likely death. Sitting next to this man, on the bench in the back of the rig, was a California highway patrol officer. The officer had a notebook and a pen and was writing as fast as he could. There were tears streaming down his face. The patient was dictating letters to his wife and children. He was hard to understand because of the swelling that was rapidly consuming his mouth and airway. However, even though he needed to be intubated quickly, nobody stopped him from what was likely the last time he would ever speak.

After finishing the letter to his wife, he moved on to his son. Nobody, except those in the back of that ambulance, can begin to understand the weight of the situation that was unfolding, and the act of immense kindness and service being performed by a highway patrol officer. The deep sense of tragedy was on the faces of everyone present. When the dictation was over, the patient's airway was too swollen for intubation, and a field surgical cricothyrotomy was performed. This means a surgical incision was made in the front of the patient's neck, and an airway was placed directly into his trachea. The patient was flown to the burn center, where he was transferred to the care of the burn team. The hospital was prepared for him. They are one of only a few burn centers in southern California capable of handling burns this serious. Unfortunately, the reason they were prepared was because they had lots of practice. They were also prepared for the wife and children who would soon arrive. A huge team of efficient medical staff swarmed the patient on arrival. There were also clergy, a social worker, and volunteers ready to accept the family when they arrived. They were prepared to make the family as comfortable as they could through this situation and the anguish they were about to face. The emergency burn team transferred the patient to the burn ICU. Then they went back to work. After the patient was dropped off at the hospital, the flight crew went back to work. After transcribing letters to the patient's family members, the highway patrol officer went back to work.

No debriefing.

No offer of assistance.

The unique thing about the previous incident is I was on the leadership side. I was not on this call. My flight crew told me all about it in great detail. I was the one who did not offer assistance. I did not hold a debriefing. As I remember, they told me the story with some understandable emotion. I honestly think my only response was something like, "Damn, that sucks." I wish I could go back and have a do-over. I wish I could look my crew in the eyes and ask them how they were doing. I would often hug my crew members when I greeted them. I wish I could go back and hug them after they shared the details of this call with me. I wish I could offer them some compassion and, perhaps, assistance if they felt they needed it.

GIVING THE BAD NEWS

One of the most stressful tasks in healthcare is informing family members of a terrible injury or the death of their loved one. It is easy to get lost in the tasks of taking care of a critical patient at times and not think about the human side of what we are doing. However, when the dust settles and the patient is stabilized or deceased and the excitement of the moment is over, that human side of things often comes rushing back to the forefront. Informing family members is a difficult task. Trying to locate family members who have no idea there has been an accident can be extremely stressful. It can also be stressful when you realize there is nobody to call for a patient because the patient hasn't anyone who seems to care about them.

Two Seventeen-year-old Boys

It was a typical Saturday in the ER. The volume of patients in this particular ER was high. Moreover, we had an unusually high number of very sick patients. In the late morning, we received two very critical patients. Both were young men, seventeen years old. One was covered from head to toe in green tattoos. Many were artistic, and many were symbols of the gang he ran with and of the life he was involved in. This young man was involved in a fight that turned into a shoot-out and was shot several times in the upper torso. When he arrived, our trauma room was already occupied by another trauma. The new patient was taken to a regular treatment room with very little space. He went into cardiac arrest just before we got him to the room.

Typically, traumatic full arrests have an extremely slim chance of survival. However, if the trauma is from penetrating wounds, as in gunshots, the patient has a greater chance of survival. Still very slim, but better than with blunt force trauma. We worked this patient up for a while and tried everything we could; however, he was too badly injured and did not survive. At the end of the shift, the staff were still unable to locate any family members for this young man, and there was no one at the hospital, besides staff, there for him.

I was not the primary nurse for the first seventeen-year-old. But I was for the second young man coming to us by helicopter. He arrived shortly after the first patient died. When this young man arrived, we learned he was the same age as the gunshot victim. His name was Brian, like mine. However, as we learned later, this young man had a strong family who loved and supported him. He was the student body president of his high school. He was an all-star volleyball player. He was a youth leader in his local church. By all accounts, he had a life that was the polar opposite of the first teen. However, trauma and illness are no respecters of persons.

We learned this young man was spending the day at the local dam. There was a small lake there where swimmers and fishermen went, and this young man and his friends were swimming. They decided to swim from one side of the lake to the other. It was a hot summer day. The water was cold but not frigid. This young man was reported to be a strong swimmer. As this group of friends began to swim across the lake, all seemed well. When they reached the halfway point, my patient began to fall behind. He eventually called out to his friends that he was in trouble.

One of his friends was only fifteen feet away from him. As the friend turned to help his buddy, he reported that Brian simply "went under the water." The remaining group of friends rushed to the scene. They all began diving in the spot where the teen went under. However, as hard as they tried, they could not find Brian. Someone on the shore had been watching. This was in the days before cell phones. That person rushed to the ranger station and called for help.

A rescue helicopter arrived in approximately twenty minutes. Their diver was able to locate Brian in another ten. It had been thirty minutes since he went underwater, and he was in cardiac arrest. Because the water was cold, they worked him up and brought him to us. Once again, our team valiantly tried everything we could to save this young man's life. We were not successful.

After he was pronounced dead, I began the task of trying to locate his family. At the time, this ER did not have a full-time social worker. This meant it was the nurses' responsibility to call family members and accompany the physician when the family received updates. This included telling family members of a loved one's passing. I obtained a home phone number and called. I can almost recall the conversation verbatim, remembering it as if it were yesterday.

"Hello," said a woman.

"Is this Mrs. Smith?" (Not her real last name.)

"Yes, it is."

"Hi, ma'am. This is Brian from the emergency room. Do you have a son named Brian Smith?"

"Yes, I do. Is everything okay?"

"Brian is here in the ER, and we need you to come down."

"Is everything okay?"

"How far away are you?"

"Five minutes. Tell me why Brian is in the ER."

"Mrs. Smith, why don't you just come down here, and we will tell you all about it."

"Is Brian okay?"

"He was in an accident at the lake and was brought to us very sick. Please do not rush while driving, but you should leave now to come here."

"I just need to get the rest of the groceries out of the car, and I will be down."

"Please be careful, but come as soon as you can. When you get here, ask for me. I will come and get you and bring you back."

It was a very difficult call. I certainly did not want to lie to her on the phone, but I also did not want to tell her that her child was dead on the phone either. Not very long after my call, I was told she was at the front desk. I went to the waiting room and met her. As we were walking back, she asked me again, "Is Brian okay?" I told her we were taking her to a quiet room, and I would go get the doctor and be right back to talk with her. As we walked to the quiet room, it really struck me that we walked right past the room where her teenage son's body lay lifeless.

I went to get the ER doctor, and we headed for the quiet room. We walked to the room and stopped outside. The doctor, one of the best I have ever worked with, asked me if I wanted to tell her or if I wanted him to. I put my hands out in front of me, my right hand with the palm up and my left fist on top. He did the same. Yes, we did rock-paper-scissors to determine who would be the one to tell her. I lost. I had listened to many different colleagues share this type of news with family members. I had my prepared statement, which I thought was the kindest way to tell them. It may not be the best, but it is how I approached the situation.

The doctor and I entered the room, and I introduced the physician to the mother of my patient. We sat down, and I wasted no time. I first asked her if she knew Brian and his friends were up at the dam. She said she did. I recounted the story we were told about them swimming across, and then Brian becoming strained and going under. I told her about the call for help and the helicopter coming and the divers rescuing him. I then told her he did not have a pulse, so the paramedics began CPR. I asked her if she understood how critically ill he was. She did.

My style of telling this to the family is an attempt to let them start figuring out where I am going. It also gives me a chance to read their reception of the information. I continued, "Brian was brought to us, and his heart was still not beating, nor was he breathing. We took over care and continued CPR." I remember how emotionless her face seemed to be. I try not to say the words "died," "deceased," "passed away," etc. I try to make a difficult thing not sound cold, partly to ease the delivery but also to make it sound less like this is something routine and we just went through the motions. I want her to know how seriously we take this and how much effort we put into trying to save her son.

Continuing, I said, "A large team, including the best doctor, nurses, and techs in the entire valley, was surrounding his bed doing everything possible to save his life. . . . However, ultimately, we were not successful." At this, I said nothing and let it sink in. She just stared off between the ER doc and me. Eventually, the doctor asked her, "Do you understand what Brian is telling you?" She looked at him and said, "He is telling me that my Brian is dead." She then looked at me—just staring at me. Eventually, her eyes welled up, and tears began streaming down both cheeks. So did mine!

The doctor offered his condolences and left the room. He was also emotional. I asked her if there was someone I could call for her. She told me her husband was at work and gave me the number. She also gave me the number of their pastor. I called the pastor, and he answered. I explained the situation to him. Thankfully, he knew them well and also knew where the patient's father worked. He said he would go to the father's place of employment and tell him personally, and then drive him to the ER.

What did I do? I went back to work. So did the doctor and the rest of the team.

No debriefing.
No offer of assistance.

I have often thought of that day. Both lives had gone in different directions. One very troubled boy, with no family support, who lived a hard, violent life. The other was just the opposite. Yet here they were, in my ER, lying fifteen feet apart, separated only by a wall. Both were very different, yet both were just as dead. I could not help but think how not that many years ago, both were little boys running and playing without a care in the world. I remember looking at the closed exam room doors, each with a dead teenager behind it. The ER was packed with patients and family members, and none of them knew of the tragedy we had just witnessed.

Just a note: The previous incident taught me a valuable lesson and caused me to develop a different approach. What I should have done, and have done since, was have the sheriff's department send a car over to the patient's house and bring the mother to the ER. Having her drive was unwise.

NONCLINICAL STRESSORS

Nursing is a rather unique profession. In most professions, if service is not provided appropriately, the business, not the employee, is responsible for making it right, if they so choose. However, as a nurse, you are a licensed professional. This means you are responsible for your own practice. I am not suggesting healthcare organizations are not responsible for the care provided and the safety of patients. They are. They also may be liable in cases of neglect, harm, malpractice, etc. However, the nurse is personally responsible and can also be held liable, civilly and criminally. Hospitals are a business. It is reality. Even those that are "not for profit" or "nonprofit." Were they not conducted as a business, they would not be able to financially support the care they provide. They must be efficient with resources and careful about waste. Most businesses have customers. Though there are some things unique about each customer, for the most part, it is all the same. A moviegoer buys a ticket, gets a snack, and is directed to their correct theater to sit down. An airline passenger buys a ticket, goes through security, boards the plane, sits down, and is flown to their destination.

In healthcare, each patient is very different: the care they receive, the resources they need, the time required to treat them, the urgency needed to address their problem, the cost of their care, etc. Sometimes (many in my profession would argue it is more), hospital administration gets so focused on the big picture, they forget we are dealing with patients—actual human beings. They look at things like "best practices" and forget every practice cannot be applied equally to every patient in every situation. They look at data and statistics and numbers and forget things like emotion, tragedy, culture, personal situations, and unique circumstances, which go into every patient encounter.

Those in nursing administration have a terrible habit of promoting individuals into leadership roles but never teaching them how to lead. Nursing is also a profession where the "alphabet soup" behind your name seems a better indicator of your ability to manage than your attitude and experience. Clinical degrees are not business or leadership degrees. And no degree can replace experience. In my view, most nursing "leaders" become the very people they complained about while they were working the floors.

Nursing is also a profession big on meetings. The leaders are continually going to meetings rather than spending time in their departments getting a feel for the employees who fall within their stewardship. Nursing tends to have more committees and subcommittees than any other profession. These committees are always coming up with "great" new ideas to implement in the hospital and individual departments. Lots of cute little "feel good" ideas that sound great in theory but rarely work in practice.

Conversely, the hospitals I have worked in do very little actual quality improvement. In healthcare, "quality," in practice, is measured by meeting national patient safety goals and CMS standards, rather than improving the practice of the individual nurses at the point of care. Skill sets of nurses are developed individually and rarely monitored. Nurses are expected to live up to the expectations of the organization, yet virtually nothing is done to measure competency and build education around deficiencies. Nurses are the first to be blamed when something goes wrong with a patient's care; however, little effort is put into ensuring the nurses are actually capable of meeting the expectations of the organization.

Education in nursing has become focused more on renewing certifications and teaching about the latest national standard, rather than helping nurses be better at their craft. All this leaves many nurses feeling inadequate and unappreciated. It drives a wedge between leadership and the staff.

Nurses are also very good at "eating their own," especially their younger, newer colleagues. This seems to be worse in the emergency department. ER nurses have a reputation for being the badasses of healthcare. The cases range from a splinter someone cannot get out to a sucking chest wound or a stroke or a child with a tummy ache. As my friend Dr. Mark Brown says in his book *Emergency!*, "We never know what the doors will bring." Patients come in, and we know very little or nothing about what happened to them. If nurses are tough, ER nurses are solid steel. Unfortunately, most ER nurses do not see this as a reputation, but rather an expectation. And most ER nurses do everything they can to live up to it.

It is remarkable to me how many nurses will swell with pride when they hear nurses "eat their young." This is a phrase that applies to many people and groups. However, nurses seem to have a special expertise in this area. Some might think the target of this is new nurses. This could not be further from the truth. In nursing, especially in the ER, nurses target new staff to the department, even if they are seasoned nurses. In my experience, this seems to mostly come from a position of insecurity. I have personally experienced this when I took on a new job.

I came to one ER, and though I was a seasoned nurse, I did not know the logistics of the ER. I was unfamiliar with some processes and had no idea where anything was. There were nurses who would not give me the time of day. Then, one day, a sick patient came in, and I took the initiative, knowing what needed to be done. Some nurses summarily dismissed my suggestions and literally pushed me out of the way. I was not trying to overstep anyone. Often in emergency care, the first person with an idea of what to do either speaks up or just gets busy. This may be the nurse or the tech or the provider. Good teams just get behind each other and do what needs to be done, regardless of the alphabet soup behind their name. Solid nurses and providers will just fall in and get to work. As the situation unfolds, the provider will take charge clinically, verify approval of what care and interventions are underway, and give clinical direction on how to proceed.

In the current example, the nurses who dismissed my input didn't consider what I was doing. They just seemed put off that the "new guy" was the one taking the initiative. I would later find these were some of the least experienced nurses in that ER. One apologized to me after she got to know me and realized my experience level. She and I discussed her approach to me. She was brave enough to be honest and admitted she was trying to look impressive to me. She was a good nurse, but for some reason, she felt threatened by a nurse she did not know and who was not asking her what to do. Once she got to know me, she realized I love to help and teach newer nurses, as well as learn the things they have an edge on. I have nothing to prove to them, and they eventually relaxed. However, this is something the "new nurse" faces every day.

Part of the insecurity comes from the culture of not wanting to look weak. This is the very culture that has fostered a climate allowing stress to build in many of my colleagues. Some nurses are insecure in their own abilities but feel the need to hide it. It is like a cancer in the industry, which adds to the stress. There is also an air with some individuals who are so determined to show everyone who is the head cock in the henhouse, they will compromise patient care to do so.

In many areas of healthcare, there is often a disconnect between providers (nurse practitioners, doctors, physician assistants, etc.) and nursing staff. I do not believe this is the case with most providers, and it is even more rare in the ER. However, it is a real problem. It also occurs between nurses and nurses' aids. I am referring to the times when those who have a higher scope of medical authority believe this makes them superior to those with a lesser scope of practice. Some feel those with lesser credentials are less professional than they are or feel they are there to serve them. Some feel those below them clinically work for them and must do as they say in all things.

Sit Down and Shut Up

It was a typical day in the small critical-access hospital I was contracted with as a travel nurse. We were patient-free at the time, and one of the members of the upper administration came to the department. I was engaged in conversation with the medical provider for the day, one of our physician assistants (PA). This provider and I had always had a good working relationship. We discussed many topics, and I thought we worked very well together.

The admin person began having a whispered conversation with the other nurse. After a short time, the admin person walked out of the department.

The nurse walked over and said she was going to do an EKG on this admin person. I asked if he was having chest pain. She said the complaint was chest tightness and shortness of breath. The PA said, "I don't want to know about this. [The admin] confided in the nurse, and it is between them." This was quite surprising, but it likely referred to the fact all chest pain patients were to be brought straight back to a room for an EKG. Since we were empty, I asked, "Why don't we bring this person right back to a bed for the EKG?" The provider then asked if this person was checking in. The nurse said, "Yes." I persisted and reminded them it was standard care and best practice to bring any patient with this type of complaint directly in for a STAT 12-lead EKG, and we should have admitting come do the registration at the bedside. The provider looked at me and told me, "Stay out of it!"

Now, I understand how things work. The provider has the final say clinically when there is a scope of practice decisions to be made! However, the provider is not always correct. Many times, they order the wrong medication for the wrong patient. It is human nature to make mistakes. Nurses are not supposed to just follow orders blindly; they are supposed to follow appropriate orders. There was no conflict whatsoever on what clinical interventions needed to be done. This was a logistics, timing, and policy conflict. In this case, the patient was having chest tightness.

The policy at this hospital, and every other ER I know of, was to bring individuals with this complaint straight back for an EKG. As previously stated, this is a best practice. Typically, orders and their timing are directed by the provider. However, nurses are compelled to ignore orders that are immoral, illegal, or unsafe. This was clearly a potential danger to the patient and against the standard of care and hospital policy. The order to stay out of it was not a clinical order and was completely out of line. The other nurse said, "I am not sure what to do." I do not believe she was referring to a clinical decision. She knew what the patient needed. We all did. She was referring to conflicting suggestions from the provider and me.

I was quite surprised by how nonchalant the provider was about letting the patient walk to the waiting room and be registered before coming back for an EKG. Again, our ER was completely void of patients at the time. The other nurse went for the EKG machine and took it to the room where we would bring the patient, and I got up and headed for the waiting room to get the patient. At this point, the PA told me, "Leave it alone. Sally (the other nurse, and not her real name) is taking care of it." I told him I was just going to get the patient for her. The PA persisted and said, "Stay out of it. Sally is handling it!"

I should have ignored him and gotten the patient, but Sally finally said she was going to get him. I turned and walked toward the PA, who was sitting in his chair, and said, "I don't work for you, and you are completely wrong!" I went back to my workstation as the PA said, "I am the provider, and one of my nurses from my ER is already taking care of the patient." Again, forgetting I could take the high road by exercising my right to remain silent, I said, "Your ER? This is all *our* ER." He said, "I am the provider, and you cannot run an ER without a provider, so it is my ER." I replied, "You cannot run an ER without nurses either. It is all our

ER." He then stunned me by saying, "Yes, you can. You don't need nurses to run an ER. It has been done before." With this, I finally turned back to my computer and said, "Wow, we have reached a new level of arrogance today."

I must admit, I have never, in my entire career, heard a provider say something so arrogant and demeaning. I was astonished. After the dust settled, I was angry with myself for not just keeping my mouth shut and doing what I knew was right for the patient. I should have ignored his directive to stay out of it. The patient should have been brought back, in spite of the provider's insane protest. With legit chest pain patients, we always swarm them to get things rolling. I failed the patient by not dismissing the provider and being a patient advocate. I failed my colleague by not setting an example of doing what is right. I failed everyone present by engaging in an immature exchange with the provider to fuel my ego instead of focusing on what was appropriate and taking care of the patient.

As a legal nurse, I assure you, had there been a poor outcome with this patient, the provider would have been completely exposed. Had the delay caused any harm to the patient, it would have been a slam-dunk case for the patient. Unfortunately, since I knew what the correct thing to do was, morally, clinically and legally, and I had the experience to understand this was a situation to ignore the provider, I would have also been guilty of contributing to the harm of the patient. Thankfully, for all of us, the patient had a good outcome, and all was well.

At the end of the day, I attempted to speak with the provider. I asked if I could explain my perspective and then allow him to explain his so we might be able to exchange ideas and hopefully move on from this in a positive way. He agreed. However, as I started to explain my side, he got angry and stormed out the door, saying, "I am not having this conversation without the department medical director present." The other nurse I was working with was completely stressed out by the situation she had witnessed.

A few days later, I was called into the manager's office with another manager present. You see, true to form in nursing, it was assumed I was in the wrong and needed disciplinary counsel. Even nurse leadership jumps to the side of the higher clinical scope of practice and assumes the nurse is in the wrong. As I explained my perspective on the situation, both nursing managers had stunned looks on their faces. It certainly seemed to be a wild tale. No reasonable person could even imagine it happened the way I explained it. I told them, as an experienced manager, I knew they needed to take what I said with a grain of salt. I asked them to please speak with the provider, and I was happy to have a meeting in person with him, the medical director, and my manager. In fact, I insisted, as it is the only real way to get to the bottom of something like this without the back and forth of a "he said, she said" scenario.

The meeting was scheduled; however, after the medical director heard from my manager, the meeting was canceled. I have no idea what the outcome was with the provider. However, there was certainly tension moving forward as we worked together.

This is a pretty extreme example of conflict, considering the complete deviation from best practices and standard of care. However, it illustrates the disconnect that seems to always be looming between people with different levels of clinical scope of practice. There should have been a discussion between all of us. I know the medical director of the ER. He is an excellent doctor and a good man. However, I have to believe there was a little "circling of the wagons" going on, which is pretty standard. Had we moved forward with our meeting, one of the medical providers would have been exposed for a poor medical decision, and we certainly cannot have that happen. It prevented a good opportunity for all of us to learn. I have a very strong personality. I can seem very bossy. I am not sure if that was part of the provider's decision to push back against me. He never seemed to be one with an ego. I lost the opportunity to admit my poor approach in front of everyone and apologize for it. The other nurse should have been allowed to be part of the resolution and hear me and the provider apologize for our respective participation in the situation, which was handled poorly, and many opportunities were missed. Any underlying stress from the situation was allowed to just fester. And so it goes!

CHANGES IN HEALTHCARE

In the early 1980s, when I first entered the world of emergency services as a young EMT, things were much different. When we responded to individuals who frequently called EMS, nothing compelled us to transport them to the hospital. In fact, I remember many times hearing law enforcement tell people they would be arrested for repeatedly abusing the system if they called without a cause.

In one such incident, my colleagues responded to a man who called because he could not burp after consuming an enormous quantity of soda. This was in the middle of the night. In Los Angeles County, the number of resources dispatched to every call is a bit much. An ambulance is sent, as in most areas. However, the closest fire engine, usually with four people on it, is also sent, as is a paramedic squad with two people. Additionally, a sheriff deputy responded. This patient was given a big slap on the back from an EMT, and he belched. He was warned by the deputy not to abuse the system. All who responded went back to their stations and to bed, except the deputy, who continued his patrol.

Once I transitioned into the ER as a tech, I saw the same thing. Everyone who came in was triaged by an experienced nurse, and once they had been seen, many of these people were educated about what the emergency room was for and sent on their way to see their own doctor or go to a clinic. Things such as a paper cut, sneezing a lot, a pinky finger that has been sore for six months, inability to orgasm during sex, hair not growing fast enough on a child, hiccups for a month, an ant bite a week ago and someone saying they might have rabies, smelly farts, smelly feet, and the list goes on and on and on.

After I became a newly trained triage nurse, I had a man come in who told me he had a rash on his "gonies." Based on where he was pointing, I assumed he meant his testicles, and he confirmed this. When I asked him how long he had had this rash, he replied, "Well, four . . . no, five years now." This was at 3 a.m. in the middle of an insanely busy shift. Exacerbated, I slammed my hand down on the desk and said, "You are telling me you have had a rash on your ball sack for five years, and now, at 3 o'clock in the morning, after all this time, it is somehow an emergency? What the heck is so terrible about it now?" Without skipping a beat, he looked me in the eyes and said, "Man, that shit just ain't going away!" I was tired and frustrated and a little amused. I did not have the energy to throw him out. I quoted him in the "chief complaint" section of my triage form and told him to go sit down, and he would likely not see a provider for six to eight hours. However, I could have kicked him out of the ER, and there would have been no repercussions for doing so, as this was clearly not an emergency.

During the same time, primary care was quite different. Many times, people would come to the ER with real complaints, albeit not emergencies. Once triaged, they were sent to registration, where they took their insurance information. Most insurances, at the time, required the primary care provider (PCP) of the patient to authorize a visit to the ER. Quite often, the patient's PCP would tell the registration clerk to have the patient leave and come to the doctor's office in the next couple of days. Even when a patient would come in for a true emergency, like a laceration requiring sutures, many times, their doctor would instruct us to send the patient right over to their office.

The entire system seemed geared toward making certain the patient received the most appropriate care and keeping the emergency room to just "emergencies." Over the years, the system has evolved, or devolved, into a completely different culture.

We live in a fast-food society where people have become accustomed to instant results. If someone feels they need to see a doctor, they often do not even try to make an appointment with one in the office. They just drive to the ER. If they do try to see their doctor and cannot get in the same day or week, they just drive to the ER. Once at the ER, just like when they go for a snack at their favorite fast-food hangout, they expect drive-through service. Gone are the days when many parents would take care of illnesses of their children at home or be patient and let an illness run its course.

When I was a kid, if I had a stuffy nose and cough, my mother would make me chicken soup and comfort me until I felt better, often in about a week. If I were vomiting, a bucket was placed next to my bed, and I was encouraged to drink plenty of water so there was "something to throw up," and I would not just have the dry heaves. Again, I was comforted until the illness ran its course. These days, parents rush their child to the ER if they vomit one time or wake up with a runny nose and sneeze or cough. If a person has diarrhea when they wake up in the morning, they often immediately come to the ER. The culture has changed to one of needing instant gratification or a remedy for anything that ails people.

The culture change in which people feel the need to rush to the ER because they feel someone needs to do something for their ailment immediately is not, by itself, a problem. The world of reimbursement has also changed and caused administration and provider groups to shift their priority focus. A portion of reimbursement is tied to "patient satisfaction." This is one of those things, in my opinion, that does not, in theory, even make sense. The word "satisfaction" in healthcare is synonymous with happiness and joy. If it meant "quality patient outcomes" in the face of competent care and the best-case scenario under the circumstances, it might make sense. However, it has come to mean "the customer is always right."

I have worked in ERs where patients and family members complain about some of the pettiest things, like the TV does not work in the room or there is no TV at all. There is no food for them, or there's no quality food. Patients with a runny nose or a cut finger will complain because we took a patient ahead of them who was being carried in and turning blue from not breathing, but "I was here first." People will call an ambulance and think that gets them in faster, then they are mad because we have the ambulance take them to the waiting room to be triaged like everyone else. Some patients who have been in the waiting room for several hours will actually leave and call 911. An ambulance will pick them up and bring them in, only to be told to take them back out to the waiting room to start all over again. (Yes, this really happens.)

Many nurses get very irritable about the definition of what is an acceptable reason to come to the ER for many people. In my observation, this is for two reasons. First, ER staff are exacerbated by people not taking any initiative to try and fix their own ailments. It is quite remarkable, some of the trivial reasons people think require a visit to the ER. Another reason, which will not sit well with some of my colleagues, is arrogance. I know many people in my business who believe some things are beneath them. They feel their time is being wasted on such trivial matters. All they believe they should be seeing are trauma and gravely ill patients. Many colleagues I interviewed have admitted this. This attitude, mixed with the compulsion by managers to make everyone happy so they do not complain, can be toxic.

SILLY COMPLAINTS

All patient complaints are reviewed and taken seriously. I believe they should be, initially. However, even the most ridiculous complaints are given time and attention to mitigate negative hits to the overall patient satisfaction score of the hospital so the insurance companies do not withhold money.

Most often, the administration will require the staff to account for the complaint. If there is a legitimate complaint about care or neglect, I am all for accountability. But when emergency staff are counseled about a person who had to wait to be seen for their minor problem because more serious patients were being tended to, it crosses a line and feeds the toxic culture.

Sometimes a patient will complain, and the complaint is so ridiculous, it should have been immediately dismissed. However, those in positions of authority often are so quick to address the staff, they do not do basic due diligence and investigate the situation.

Paranoid

I had a certain patient who came in on a particular shift with some type of complaint. I do not even remember what it was. I do remember when we told him each time it was not serious, he added another complaint. He desperately wanted something to be wrong; however, it was just not meant to be. He was physically very healthy.

One day, my shift was interrupted by a supervisor who wanted to speak with me. The charge nurse covered my patients, and I went to "the office." The supervisor asked me about the above patient. She told me the patient felt I was not compassionate, saying that "My nurse made it clear he did not like me." He made the same charge against the ER doctor. I laughed out loud. I asked the supervisor if she had looked at the chart and the patient's history. She admitted she had not. I told her this patient had an active diagnosis of paranoid schizophrenia. He thinks everyone hates him and is out to get him.

Despite telling her this and the doctor defending my manner with the patient, I was counseled and given a sheet of paper with ideas to better interact with difficult patients. I was amused but also angry. At that time, I had more complimentary letters from patients and families than anyone in my department. I could not believe this patient's complaint was given this much effort and attention.

Staff feel pressure to hurry and deal with the life-threatening issues quickly so the patients with minor emergencies or nonemergencies won't get mad and complain to management because it took too long. Most repeat patients who abuse the system and the staff know their satisfaction will be a factor. Often, they tell the staff this in real time and threaten to give them a poor evaluation. This adds to the stress. For some, it manifests itself as anger and disgust toward nearly all patients and their family members. For others, it creates tremendous stress as they try to be all things to all people while worrying they will get in trouble if they fail.

Imagine how stressful a typical good day in healthcare is. Good practitioners are always mindful of how a mistake could adversely affect another human being. Even when someone is being treated for a stuffy nose, the staff wonders if they missed something or if it was really a simple issue. I am not suggesting we worry about and ponder every little decision. I am simply pointing out the thoughts are there. Consider how stressful it becomes when a true emergency is encountered. A patient presents with a life-threatening issue where a lack of immediate action by the staff will mean certain death. In the ER, these things often happen without warning.

Fentanyl

On a particular day while I was working in a critical-access hospital emergency department, we were unusually busy with multiple critical patients at the same time. We had a patient who was leaving by helicopter for a critical care unit for a serious diabetic problem, and there was another patient with a serious active bleeding issue whose helicopter crew had just arrived to get him. Another patient had recently arrived by ambulance with uncontrolled seizures and was being prepared to possibly be intubated and placed on a ventilator.

I have worked in many hospitals where this is just another day and frankly, not a big deal. Most ER staff reading this will likely shrug their shoulders if they have not worked in a small, critical-access ER, which typically staffs just two RNs, a tech, and a provider. And we had a very small number of inpatient medical beds for stable patients who required observation and minimal intervention. However, because we had several critical patients that day, we had two nurses from the medical floor who came to offer some extra hands.

While we were handling our business, I received a call from the front desk and was told there was a patient outside in the car who was choking. I have learned not to believe anything I hear when it is reported to me. It is rarely accurate information. I pay attention and look into the problem; however, I do not assume I am getting the real story. Most of my experienced colleagues would certainly agree.

I headed out to the front to see what the issue was. A few of the extra staff who came to help in the ER went with me. I asked one to bring a wheelchair in case we needed it. When I walked out the front door toward the parking lot, a man frantically waved to me and said, "Hurry, he is turning blue!" As I got to the car, I could see the man was mistaken.

The patient was not blue; he was gray. This is worse!! His lips were blue, but the rest of his skin was a dusky gray color, which meant he was almost dead. He was slumped forward in the passenger seat of the car. I grabbed hold of his upper body and picked him up out of the car. Someone else took his legs, and we placed him in the wheelchair.

The man who brought him said they had just left a restaurant, and his friend began "choking," so he drove straight to the hospital. I pulled the patient's head back to open his airway, and there was a gasping sound. That was a relatively good sign. We wheeled him into the hospital and to the ER. When we placed him on the gurney, his color had improved slightly.

We have amazing air medical crews, and one of the flight nurses who was there to get the bleeding patient came to the bedside to assist us. As IVs were established and the respiratory team was assisting the patient's breathing, the provider called for Narcan. This is a medicine that reverses the effects of narcotics. It is harmless if given to someone without needing narcotic reversal, and it is a good option in an unknown situation like this, especially in the community I am referring to.

While getting the Narcan ready and waiting for IV access, the provider used a laryngoscope to visualize the airway, since the patient's friend said he was choking on something. The airway was clear, the respiratory team was getting good ventilation with the bag, and the patient's color was back to normal. But he was still not breathing and was completely unresponsive.

Please consider the entire situation. Prior to this man's arrival, we were already busy and completely maxed out on our resources. We had multiple critical patients requiring our attention, and then this patient, who needed immediate attention for survival. One could argue we could not handle another crisis until we purged some of what we had. However, not only did we get another sick patient, but we were presented with a patient who required us to drop what we were doing to save his life. Literally!!

During this time, there were several patients in the waiting room with non-life-threatening issues who had to wait, and nobody complained; however, I present this scenario to illustrate what happens in the ER. It is in situations just like this where people often complain about the wait. Any reasonable person who hears this story would agree we were prioritizing our resources appropriately, but in nearly every hospital I have worked in, if a patient with a splinter in their pinky toe complained about the wait, in this exact situation, the staff would have to account for the complaint. In most cases, they would be required to explore what they could have done differently and if there was any way they could have gotten to the toe problem faster. Incidentally, the "choking" patient was given the Narcan and was wide awake and alert within sixty seconds, having consumed street fentanyl.

In this scenario, it is easy to see how the staff, in many hospitals, may feel pressured to rush through their care of the patient who is not breathing so they do not get in trouble if a patient in the waiting room complains. This is a serious issue and adds a tremendous level of stress to the staff. It is common for sudden emergencies to happen and for multiple staff members to enter the room, perform tasks, then leave when no longer needed. Perhaps they start an IV, get vital signs, get the patient undressed, assist with ventilations until respiratory arrives, etc.

Even routine help when we "swarm" a patient carries with it the thoughts of inadequacy. "What am I dropping to come do this?" "How far behind am I going to be on my charting now?" "I left meds on the counter to come in here. I hope nobody picks them up." "I almost wet my pants because I have not been able to get to the bathroom, and now I cannot even think straight while I am bagging this patient." All are real concerns and are typical of the emergency room. Most of these things cannot be helped and are just part of the job.

I am not suggesting anything can be done to prevent this type of thing from happening. However, they are real stressors contributing to the overall burden of the staff. When the consideration of these circumstances seems to be ignored by the administration as they look at patient satisfaction scores, it creates a real feeling of being dejected among the staff. For the record, in the ER, where the above situation happened, the manager is a rock star and does not forget what the staff are encountering at the bedside.

PEER PRESSURE

Peer pressure is another huge factor in the toxic culture. Earlier, I discussed how the example we set of not showing emotions is hereditary in the family of emergency services. While I rarely see those who are senior staff express emotions, there are other experienced people who actively campaign to prevent it.

I was working CCT (critical care transport) and was stationed at the same base with a 911 ambulance crew. They had a new EMT hire. The medic, a salty, experienced guy, was sharing a story of a time when another new EMT was on a call with him. There was a death in the house they responded to. The new EMT was outside crying after the call was over. This experienced medic was laughing and telling everyone, "That chick is never going to make it in this business. She was already crying before she was finished with her orientation."

This attitude is exactly the problem. The other new EMT who was present for the story felt compelled to laugh at what was being said. The climate was already being set for her to be afraid of speaking up when something was bothering her. I spoke up and said there was nothing wrong with being human, and the only thing required in our line of work is to be able to function in the moment.

We are called on to help people in tragic situations and need to be able to complete our tasks. Of course, this takes some time to be able to temper our emotions and focus on our job. Making fun of people for having real human emotions is counterproductive to an emotionally healthy workforce. Additionally, as long as someone is able to function in their job duties, there is nothing wrong with expressing their emotions after the fact. That is exactly the time to begin the debriefing session, as some will become emotionally affected in the moment and not be able to effectively complete the task at hand.

Though this is something that can affect the care being provided and should be addressed immediately, it is not anything that should be viewed as abnormal or detrimental to the career of the individual. Some people will be able to vent right after the call and move on. Others may need to seek the help of a third party to help them work through their emotions.

In all cases, everything should be done to help the individual remain productive. Making fun of and mocking the caregiver should never happen. It is important not to foster a culture where it is cool to make fun of people who express their emotions.

SUPPLIES AND EQUIPMENT

Budget is a sensitive subject among my colleagues. I understand administrations need to focus on "the bottom line." It usually surprises my colleagues when I tell them the bottom line must come ahead of quality patient care, overall. Let me explain. If a hospital is not profitable, no patient care will take place. It is that simple. Though it is healthcare, and we are in the business of taking care of people, we must have resources to do it. I'm not going to get into a political discussion in this book. However, even in socialized healthcare systems, profitability is paramount. Any organization must be able to watch expenses, or they will be out of the healthcare business.

I am simply pointing out that a healthcare organization needs to make more than it is spending. That is simple economics. However, even though I believe financial responsibility is most important, quality patient care cannot suffer in the process. Often, it seems the pressure from the corporate office for management to be fiscally responsible is translated to mean it is the only thing that matters. I have worked for a few managers who refuse to let their staff "work with broken equipment." In industry, it is a given that quality production requires quality resources and working equipment. This concept seems to be lost in healthcare. It is astonishing how profound this problem is. I cannot think of a single hospital I have worked in where the staff was not working with broken stuff. Not a single facility. I believe it is a leadership problem. Managers in healthcare grew up in a business where working with broken stuff was the norm.

In the ER, especially, it seems dealing with catastrophe and improvising is a badge of honor. Therefore, working around problems is the norm. This includes working around broken equipment. Additionally, the culture seems to be one of never getting things fixed, so the staff gives up and puts their effort into working around it, rather than demanding it be fixed.

Often, staff are in an exam room, trying to take a blood pressure or get an otoscope to the provider, etc., and it does not work. In an already busy environment, this frustrates the staff and contributes to stress. I worked in a very prestigious and wealthy academic hospital with poor management. We did not have IV poles in the rooms. In most emergency rooms, there are ceiling IV poles. If not, all ER gurneys have IV poles attached. In this particular ER, nearly all the gurneys did not have working IV poles. There were no mounted poles in the rooms. Nurses were rigging makeshift hangars from miscellaneous supplies to the exam lights in the room. It was unbelievable how this place did not have the basic tools to do the job. The staff was so good at rigging their own, it was something taught to new employees during their department orientation. This is just one example of nonsense we dealt with in that ER. Staff all over the world seem to be great at workarounds. It is no wonder we have all learned to just deal with our own emotions as well.

SET UP FOR FAILURE

A myth exists in healthcare that says, "The person with the highest scope of practice rules the rest." This is not true. There is certainly an established hierarchy involving "scope of practice." This most often means the provider orders an intervention, and the nurse executes the intervention. However, it is not as simple as it sounds. Every nurse is compelled to question the intervention if there is confusion regarding its necessity, or if the nurse feels it is immoral, illegal, or unsafe. This can be a slippery slope when there is an emergency, and a timely intervention is necessary. Even in time-critical situations, the nurse must be confident the provider's order is safe.

This is a profoundly stressful position for nurses to be in. The nurse is a licensed professional and not a robot. Nurses are liable for what they do and allow to be done to patients. They must be the patient's advocate first. If they execute an incorrect order, they may cause harm to another human being. This is not only potentially harmful to the patient, but it can also cause the nurse to lose their job, lose their license to practice, or even face criminal charges. At the same time, if they delay an appropriate order due to ignorance, they are equally liable if they harm the patient. This is another huge stressor in nursing.

Most experienced nurses are confident enough to speak up when there is a question about an order. They have come to know most medical providers are not put off if they are asked to clarify an order and its necessity. However, many newer nurses fall into the culture of doing whatever the provider orders, regardless of their doubts. When you mix in the culture of nurses feeling like they must not look weak, disaster can follow.

Most providers in the ER are filled with confidence, and the staff sense it. Because of this, orders are rarely questioned by newer nurses. Ironically, these same providers' confidence makes them more approachable. Their confidence prevents them from taking offense when a nurse questions an order or asks why it is being given. Nearly every day, ER providers order treatments for the wrong patient. This certainly does not make them bad providers. It makes them human. We have checks and balances, and nurses must know what they are giving and why.

ER providers are constantly interrupted. Multiple nurses and techs are approaching providers with questions about various things. They are often fielding phone calls from consulting providers or making calls to other departments. The provider may be in the middle of dictating about one patient, and someone interrupts them for a question about another patient. The provider switches focus back and forth. It is very easy to conflate facts between patients. With computer charting, it is easy to click on an order but be on the wrong patient's screen. An intervention is ordered, but for the wrong patient.

Many nurses, especially new ones, execute orders every day without giving them a second thought. The vast majority of the time, it is not a factor. Giving the wrong patient Tylenol is not necessarily a big deal. However, there are times when the order will adversely affect the patient's outcome. As a nurse, I need to understand what is wrong with my patient. I need to know why everything a provider orders for my patient is being done. If I do not know, I look through the chart to see if results have come in I was unaware of. If I still do not know why something was ordered, I approach the provider and ask. I usually get an explanation from them, which satisfies my ignorance. Not infrequently, a provider will say something like, "I did not order that for Mr. Jones." After a little investigation, we realized it was ordered for the wrong patient. A correction is made, most often the provider thanks me, and we press forward. It is not a big deal, even though it could have been. If a nurse feels they are working with a provider who is not approachable, it can be disastrous. Worse yet, if a nurse feels they should know something and are afraid to ask, the outcome can be deadly.

Medication Error

While working in a leadership role at a small hospital, I was called to one of the departments regarding a med error. A medication, which was infusing into a patient, was supposed to be titrated based on blood work. A relatively new nurse was caring for this patient. It came time for the medication administration rate to be evaluated for change based on the new lab result. Unfortunately, the lab test had not been ordered, so the only result available was the result from the previous lab draw and medication change.

The nurse should have ordered a STAT lab draw and then adjusted the medication based on the new result. That would have been the end of it. However, this nurse simply adjusted the medication based on the previous result. The medication had already been adjusted to that result, which meant the new adjustment was incorrect. When the time came for the next adjustment, the blood was drawn, and the lab result was obviously way off from what was expected. It took many hours to get the lab value back to a therapeutic level.

As bad as this was, the exact same thing happened the next day. This meant the patient's blood work and body were changing wildly, and the treatment was ineffective. I was called after the second snafu. I placed a call to the admitting physician, who was understandably very upset. Corrections were made, the nurse was briefly educated, and an incident report was filed.

At the first available opportunity, I met with the department manager and explained to her the situation. I recommended this nurse be remediated and shadowed by an educator to make certain he was not in over his head. He made a serious mistake by not checking with his charge nurse when he had a question about a process he clearly did not understand. Not knowing was not the issue. This happens all the time, and advice is sought from more experienced nurses. In this case, moving forward without asking for help was the problem. My exact words to the manager were, "If someone does not help this nurse, he is possibly going to kill someone." This is a strong statement, and one I did not make lightly. The response I received from the manager stunned me. She said something like, "I know this is a problem, and we will address it. However, pulling him from the floor for remediation would be embarrassing for him. He is so sweet, and I just don't want to do that." Let that sink in. His lack of skill and critical thinking were not a problem because he was sweet and nice.

Almost to the day, a year later, my fear came true. This same nurse was caring for an elderly patient who had suffered significant orthopedic trauma. He had a very long surgery to make the necessary repairs. During the surgery, the anesthesia team gave him quite a lot of fentanyl for comfort and pain control. Fentanyl is good in this scenario because it has little or no effect on the patient's blood pressure. It does suppress respiratory drive; however, in surgery, the patient's airway and breathing are managed mechanically, so there is no issue. The half-life of the medication is short, which means it wears off pretty quickly after the last dose is given so the patient is easier to wake up after surgery. After recovery, this patient was taken to the medical and surgical floor.

In order for the fentanyl to be properly documented and billed, the pharmacy loaded it into the patient's chart. Somehow, it populated in the medication administration record and appeared as a new order to be given. The entire amount of 1200 mcg was ordered to be given. The nurse, the same one who previously did not ask for help, saw the order and went to get the medication.

This nurse had never given fentanyl. Fentanyl is very powerful and given judiciously in areas where nurses are specifically trained to give it and are familiar with it. Fentanyl is routinely given in the operating room, emergency room, and intensive care unit. It is also given in some procedural departments. However, it is never given on a regular nursing floor as an IV push; rather, it's only given in a device that restricts the administration. Other long-lasting medications are given for pain in those areas.

This nurse had no idea what he was giving and what the appropriate dosing was. When he was required to pull out twelve ampules to get the correct dose, he remembered something from nursing school. Nurses are taught if it takes more than two vials or ampules to equal the ordered dose, question the order. This nurse did pause. However, he decided to just give half the ordered dose to be safe. He correctly thought twelve ampules were too many, even though unfamiliar with the medication.

Unfortunately, for his patient, half the ordered dose of 1200 mcg is still 600 mcg, which is six times more than the maximum dose, and twenty-four times more than the standard appropriate dose for this patient. Rather than asking for clarification, even from another nurse, he drew up 600 mcg and administered it into the IV of his elderly patient. In short order, the patient slipped into respiratory and then cardiopulmonary arrest. A code blue was called, and CPR was initiated. The patient's pulse was eventually restored, and he was moved to the ICU. However, he died a couple of days later.

I share the above story for a couple of reasons. I am not certain what was going through this nurse's mind when he knowingly decided to administer medication when he had clear concerns. He later admitted he had never even given fentanyl before. I am not sure if he was completely obtuse or just did not care if there was a bad outcome. Perhaps he was terrified of looking stupid for asking questions because the culture says you have to press forward and not appear to be incompetent. Whatever the case, he demonstrated a pattern of behavior that was profoundly unsafe.

The other, more concerning issue for me has to do with the leadership of that hospital. I had warned the department manager this nurse was likely to make a catastrophic error if he was not retrained and given the proper tools to make better decisions. The department manager was more concerned with not hurting the nurse's feelings than protecting the patients and this nurse. After learning of this incident, I felt sick. I literally thought I would vomit. I immediately went to the chief nursing officer. I shared my story from the previous year and explained how I had warned the manager something like this was bound to happen if this nurse was not properly trained. She seemed concerned, and I left her office.

A few days later, I was talking to one of the doctors, who happened to be the admitting doctor of this elderly patient. He was lamenting to me about the case and then asked me a question. He said something like, "I don't really know this nurse. How could he make such an error? Do you know anything about him?" Since it was his patient, I felt he should be in the loop. I relayed the story of the previous year, where this nurse had made a terrible mistake and error in judgment. I also told him I had warned the manager about the potential for disaster if they did not intervene and give this nurse some proper education. He was flabbergasted! He then went to the hospital administration and wanted to know why this had happened.

Shortly after, I was called into the chief nursing officer's office. I was thoroughly reprimanded for sharing what I knew with this patient's doctor. It seemed to me they were circling the wagons and trying to sweep what really happened under the rug. In the end, it was determined there were many errors made, and it was a collective problem. The nurse continued to work his shifts and, to my knowledge, was never remediated.

This situation weighed heavily on me. I could not imagine what reason there would be not to share this information with the doctor of this man. Often, it seems the frontline workers are thrown under the bus as scapegoats when something goes wrong. In this case, it was a leadership problem that could not be denied by those in the know. So, it was polished over. An "error" was reported to the family. However, it was with the caveat that the error likely did not change the inevitable outcome, and the patient would have died from the original trauma. Additionally, the family was not told this same nurse had made serious errors previously and was never given proper corrective training.

While I believe the motivation to cover up what really happened was liability mitigation, it did nothing to help the nurse take corrective action. This nurse had demonstrated a pattern of not realizing the potential harm of administering medications ignorantly. He seemed to be willing to play Russian roulette with patients' lives and just hoped nothing would go wrong. We will never know if the elderly patient would have died regardless of the medication error. The nurse involved seemed to be a good person. I am sure he thinks about what he did and how it likely contributed to the death of this patient. At least, I certainly hope he does. What I do know is he was set up for failure by not being given all the tools necessary to properly do his job and make good decisions.

Though the mistake was his, it might have been averted if he had been properly remediated after the first clinical debacle.

I remain torn about not informing the patient's family about what actually happened.

BITTERNESS

There is tremendous peer pressure to "suck it up" and be tough. I see staff in the ER who seem to think the more bitter and callous they come off, the cooler and stronger they will appear to those around them. There is a dichotomy to this. Coping mechanisms are as different as the people themselves. The goal of most is to be able to detach emotionally from the personal tragedy experienced. Some do this more effectively or constructively than others. Many seem to only be able to detach by forcing their thought process to the opposite end of the spectrum from compassion. This may be why they feel it necessary to be angry at those around them.

I have seen ER staff who will speak so terribly about a patient or the family members who come to the ER. If other staff feel it crosses a line and they attempt to diffuse this attitude, often, the angry staff member turns their anger toward the helpful colleagues. It seems when someone chooses to be angry, they do not want anyone raining on their parade.

This attitude becomes a guide for others who are finding it difficult to cope with the stress of emergency services. In the absence of a productive approach to coping, they fall into something they have seen others get away with. Many times, this anger is presented comedically. This tends to get more staff on board because the attacks on the patient or family seem funny and elicit a response that is more acceptable.

Many emergency services staff get angry if they do not feel the patients presenting have a good enough reason to be in the ER. There is certainly something to be said about the abuse of the ER. Many people come for such frivolous reasons and expect the same attention as those who have real emergencies. However, staff who take it personally or allow themselves to be angered by it are simply hurting themselves. It does not change the situation by becoming upset over it. It actually contributes to the overall stress of the work environment.

This leads to a previously mentioned phenomenon where staff begin to think they should only be caring for people who "deserve" their skills and experience. Sometimes this leads to embarrassment.

Open Mouth, Insert Foot

After I had worked as a flight nurse for almost five years, I had the opportunity to be promoted to chief flight nurse (medical manager). At the time, this was a four-helicopter base operation in southern California. By the time I left the company, we had opened two additional bases. The air medical leadership, in most companies, is divided into three categories: aviation, which covers the pilots; maintenance for all mechanics; and medical, including flight nurses and flight medics. I was over the latter, and all my employees were type A hard chargers, many with far more clinical experience than I had.

One of the first things I was faced with was a complaint from a pilot and medic about a situation that occurred in the previous couple of days involving a flight nurse. The crew had been launched for a transport from one hospital to another, and the sending hospital was a quality trauma center; however, the patient required a hospital that performed organ transplant surgeries.

In air medicine, patient information is usually sparse prior to the launch. This is a safety measure. If the flight crew has too much information about the patient, they may feel compelled to take the transport when they might otherwise turn it down due to poor weather.

As they arrived at the sending facility, dispatch contacted them over the radio and advised them not to make patient contact but to call dispatch. Once the aircraft was shut down, the flight nurse called dispatch. She was informed there was an issue with the receiving facility not actually having a bed. They were to stand by until this was resolved. Since they had already accepted the flight, the dispatcher gave more detailed patient information to the nurse. This was a patient with esophageal varices from portal hypertension. This is a condition most often caused by alcoholism. The patient also had a diagnosis of pulmonary hypertension.

The nurse was extremely upset and began to rant. The pilot and medic were sitting in the helicopter with her. She started to curse and verbalize how ridiculous it was they were stuck there waiting for the transfer center to finish their jobs. She speculated how this was likely some fat, unhealthy, irresponsible slob who has been drinking his woes away all his life. He was a leech on the system and society, and he could not work because he sat around smoking and drinking all day long, ruining his health and his life. By doing so, he now caused this critical care helicopter team to waste their time by sitting around while hospitals tried to figure out who was going to take him and how to mitigate their financial losses that losers like this created for them. Her rant was wrought with profanities, and she was yelling loudly while venting all her frustrations about this terrible person who got himself into this position and did not deserve any of the effort being wasted on him.

While she was in the middle of an especially vile personal attack on this patient, she was interrupted by the voice of a man approaching the helicopter from behind. She paused and turned, asking him what he needed. He asked something like this: "Are you the crew who will be transporting my brother to Los Angeles?" The nurse, now surprised into silence, finally responded, "We will be transporting someone. Who is your brother?" The gentleman told her, and, indeed, it was the patient they were there to pick up. He graciously thanked them for the care they would be providing. He then explained how his brother, the patient, is a mechanical engineer. He was a fitness and health fanatic who ran marathons and rode 200-mile road races on his bicycle. He was a vegetarian who did not drink or smoke or do any recreational drugs. He had developed a blood-clotting issue, which caused his current disease to take a turn for the worse. Though alcoholism is the primary cause of the condition, this patient was clearly one of the exceptions. The flight nurse went out of her way to be compassionate and sound caring; however, the patient's brother had heard most of what she said and knew she was speculating about his brother.

My boss, the program director, had received a complaint from the pilot and medic. He was happy to drop it in my lap as soon as I took the reins as his chief flight nurse. The brother also contacted me to express his disappointment in what he had heard the flight nurse say. However, he was adamant about not wanting her disciplined; rather, he wanted all the crews educated about jumping to conclusions. He was remarkably understanding.

He told me he had another brother who was an ER nurse, and he knew the pressures and types of patients we were used to dealing with. His entire family had already dealt with a myriad of healthcare professionals assuming his brother was an alcoholic. I assured him I would take care of the situation and explained to him this nurse's opinion is not representative of our organization. My boss reminded me of what a terrific nurse she is. He told me this was just her being herself, and she needed to be reeled in about every six months.

A few days later, I invited the aviation manager to join me in a meeting with this nurse. We went to the base where she was working a shift, and we grounded their aircraft so we would have uninterrupted time. I asked this nurse if she remembered transporting the patient. I believe she sensed why we were there, and she began to explain the complexity of the patient and all they did to safely transport him to the receiving facility. I was impressed, but not more than usual. This is what we did every day, and her transport was no different than anyone else's.

I asked her if she remembered being upset about the transport and ranting about it to her crew. She became silent and just looked at us. I explained to her what the program director had told me. I then told her this was the only meeting like this we were going to have—that I was not going to encourage her to "reset" every six months. I told her I wanted her to be successful and knew she could be. However, I made it clear she would not be staying with our company if she had another episode like the previous one. I asked her if my message was clear to her. She acknowledged it was.

This was a solid and seasoned nurse who had been with the company long before I came along. I had flown many calls with her and knew her capabilities. She was actually one of the nurses whom I flew orientation shifts with when I was hired. I then softened my tone and asked her if there was anything we could do for her to help her or her family. This must have been the right question. She broke down and began to cry. After sobbing for some time, she shared with us some very personal things. She and her husband were struggling in their relationship because she was away from home so much. She was in school full-time, trying to complete her advanced nursing degree. We listened to her share her struggles and did what we could to offer our support while holding the line on what we had previously told her.

I wish I had known then what I have learned about stress and appropriate resources. I would have offered her more effective support.

EXACERBATION

Sometimes the staff will get to their tipping point and just go off. They will have repeated situations with the same outcome and simply get emotionally exhausted. I have seen staff members do this to patients, family members, colleagues, providers, etc. To me, this is a warning sign of something going on with the staff member. Stress had built up and had finally been released.

Too Drunk to Discharge

One night, I was working in the ER, and we had a drunk come in. There was nothing unusual about this. Sometimes, drunks will be "happy drunks" and not too difficult to deal with. This was not one of those times. This was an angry drunk, and he was being rude to the staff. I was the primary nurse. My tech was one of the best I have ever worked with. She was simply amazing. She was skilled, compassionate, and very proactive.

A term we often use in the ER is MTF. This stands for "metabolize 'til freedom." In other words, burn off enough of whatever was consumed to allow for a safe discharge. After getting our patient settled in, to let him MTF, we went about our business. A short time later, I noticed the patient trying to get up. When I went into the room, it was clear he was far too impaired to be able to sit up in the bed, let alone walk. I encouraged him to lie back down and sleep. He was mumbling something I could not understand. My tech entered the room to see if I needed any help. The patient continued to try and sit up but kept falling over in bed. We insisted he lie back down. This just made him angry. He began shouting garbled words and swinging his arms around at us. He kicked toward my tech but missed her. This made her quite angry, and she snapped. She said, "If he is awake enough to fight with us, he is awake enough to be discharged."

We put the patient in soft restraints to keep him safely in the gurney. After getting this accomplished, I went back to the nurses' station to find my tech still going on about the patient. She insisted we discharge him and made several derogatory comments about him, which I must say I did not disagree with. I continued to reason with her, trying to calm her down. She said, "Why do we coddle these assholes and allow them to treat the staff like this?" She then said, "This guy needs to be discharged to teach him a lesson that he cannot fight with the staff who are trying to help him."

One of the stressors, which is covered elsewhere in this book, is violence toward the staff. This is a very real thing and should never be taken lightly. However, though there is never an excuse for bad behavior, there are times when the unruly patient is simply too impaired to reason with and be safely discharged. In a very serious tone, I finally said to this tech, "Enough! I know he is being an asshole. However, he is not even able to sit up straight in bed. If we discharge him, he is most certainly going to fall down and hurt himself, possibly very seriously. This is unacceptable, and as a patient advocate, I cannot allow that to happen!" This stopped the rant; however, it was clear she was now even more upset with me.

It took nearly a week and a calm conversation with her to settle the air between us. I love working with her, and we are on good terms. She is one of my favorite techs. This tech did not just go off about this one situation, however. Many things were building in her, and this jerk was the spark that lit the fuse. This is one example of stress building up to a point of boiling over, being triggered by a seemingly insignificant event.

WORKPLACE VIOLENCE

Violence in the workplace is not something unique to any profession. At any time, an employee can become violent with the staff. This can happen in a flower shop, a school, a bakery, a manufacturing plant, etc. However, in healthcare, especially emergency services, violence is a regular part of the job, sometimes daily. Unfortunately, because it is something expected to happen, it is often viewed as an acceptable risk in the job. I could not disagree more.

There are certainly times when patients are out of their heads and strike out at the staff without knowing or understanding what they are doing. This happens with patients suffering from dementia, Alzheimer's, a stroke, traumatic brain injuries, Down syndrome, etc. It is something healthcare professionals train for. In cases where patients do not know what they are doing or are confused, most staff understand this and do not take it personally; however, many staff still take attacks from these types of patients personally. It is part of human nature, and it takes practice to realize it is not personal. Even when staff do not take it personally, it adds to the stress of the job when you have to physically protect or defend yourself.

In the ER, the training is more advanced. Emergency services are areas of healthcare where potential violence is exponentially higher. Though they deal with the same patient listed above, they also deal with behavioral issues unique to their area of expertise. They get patients under the influence of a wide variety of mind-altering substances. Some of these individuals can be extremely violent toward the staff; they must remain vigilant, as all of these people are potentially violent. In spite of the potential threat, the staff must get up close and personal with all patients. Just obtaining basic vital signs requires them to be in a patient's personal space, and some activities require them to be closer, such as starting an IV, drawing blood, giving an injection, or performing an EKG. These require focused attention and are times when the staff are the most vulnerable.

IV Start

I was working in the ER on a routine day. I had a male patient whom I was assigned to care for. I do not remember what he was in the ER for, but he needed an IV. He was in his thirties and a fairly large, athletic man. I remember having a pretty good rapport with him. I always talk to my patients and get to know something about them. It helps me personalize them and remember they are people. It also, most often, relaxes them and settles their nerves about being in the ER and wondering what we will be doing to them.

I explained to this gentleman what I would be doing. He never objected. I placed a tourniquet on his arm and began my routine process of finding the best vein to place the IV into. Once I found a good one, I explained to him what I would be doing and where. He said, "Okay." I prepared my supplies and cleaned his arm. I then said the same thing I always say: "Okay, great big poke coming. Please hold still."

As soon as I inserted the needle, the patient jerked his arm away from me, yelled some expletives, and swung his free arm at me with a clenched fist. Though I was in no way expecting this response, my positioning next to him allowed me to rapidly back away, avoiding the incoming strike to my head. The arm I selected was the one away from the door. This means the patient and gurney were between me and the door. The patient came up off the bed with his eyes fixed on me. He was bleeding from his arm where the needle had been. I was holding the bloody needle in my hand and was backed up against the wall.

I spotted a large male colleague walking past the door and shouted his name. He turned to look at me and immediately realized the situation I was in. I threw the bloody needle forward under the gurney so neither I nor any of the staff who would soon be coming to my rescue would get poked. I was calling the patient by name and trying to calm him. He was having none of it. As he came off the gurney toward me, he swung his blood-covered arm toward me. As he did that, I deflected the blow and turned him away from the staff member who was coming from the hall. That staff member pushed the patient toward the wall, and they both crashed into it. I jumped back into the fray and helped press the patient against the wall of the room.

Since this was a large, busy ER, several other staff had heard the commotion and were already entering the room. The patient was as strong as a bull, and the first two additional staff members helped press the patient against the wall. Other staff and a couple of security guards came into the room. We were able to secure all the patient's extremities and place him on the gurney and into restraints. It turns out this patient had a long history of mental problems, which were not apparent to me during our interactions. He had never been to our hospital before, so there was no previous history to alert us.

The above story illustrates what can happen and how it can be effectively dealt with by experienced staff. However, many hospitals are not large but small, with limited staff. If they have just two or three staff in the ER, often there is one staff member in each room and no staff in the nurses' station. If you apply the above story to most critical-access ERs, the situation becomes very different and potentially much more dangerous. It is likely—were I in a critical-access hospital for the above situation—I would have had to deal with this patient all by myself for several minutes before any of my colleagues even knew I was in trouble. I am six feet tall and in good shape. I can handle myself pretty well. However, I work in a predominantly female industry. Often, the only staff are women, and many of them are quite petite. If the story of the IV start occurred in a critical-access hospital and the staff member was a petite woman, it is easy to imagine how much danger that professional would be in.

Sometimes the violence can be anticipated and yet still be unavoidable. We have specific training in healthcare, and especially the ER, to recognize circumstances where violence is not only possible but likely. We are taught to have situational awareness. This can be difficult because we are also supposed to be in the mode of caring for the people in our charge. Caring for people and, at the same time, being suspicious of them or their visitors can be difficult. It is also difficult to know how some people will respond when we flex our authority and try to diffuse a situation that is getting out of hand.

Knockout

One day, we had a gang member who was stabbed. He was brought to the ER on a busy trauma day. As it often happens, the large trauma suite was occupied, and we had to run this trauma in a small exam room. This patient was dropped off at the ER door and was brought straight back. I was not in the room for the first part of the story. The ER

163

doctor, a nurse practitioner, and a nurse, who happened to be a guy, were in the room. A trauma code had not yet been called for some reason, so there was not an abundance of staff.

The patient had stab wounds to his chest and was in bad shape. The ER doctor was preparing to place a chest tube in the patient. While this was happening, a fellow gang member had snuck into the ER through an open door. He asked where the stab wound patient was, and an inexperienced staff member pointed him toward the room. As this guy entered the room where his "homie" was being cared for, he saw the ER doctor with a scalpel opening a hole in the patient's chest to insert the tube. This guy yelled at the doctor and told him he'd better save his homie's life or there would be hell to pay. The nurse practitioner placed her hand on this guy's shoulder and asked him if he would leave the room so they had room to work. The gang member pushed the nurse practitioner in the chest and said, "Bitch, don't put your hands on me."

With that, the male nurse pushed the gang member away from the nurse practitioner, and before he could say a word, he was knocked out cold with one punch from the gang member. The nurse practitioner screamed for help. This brought several male staff to the room. However, the gang member was prepared for a fight and started swinging. Several staff members, including me, jumped onto the gang member. Blows were flying, and punches landed on both sides of the battle line.

In the ER, we eventually produce an overwhelming number of staff to win in situations like this. To paraphrase comedian Ron White, "We did not know how many staff it was going to take to win this fight, but we knew how many we were going to use (2003)."

The gang member was quickly subdued and taken from the room to the waiting arms of the sheriff. Meanwhile, the nurse was still lying on the floor, and the ER doctor was still inserting the chest tube. The nurse was helped up after he awoke, and the doctor completed the procedure. It was almost comical. Soon, more gang members arrived, but so did more sheriff deputies. The patient died within an hour of his injuries. The gang member who knocked out the nurse, went to jail. The unlucky nurse recovered and finished his shift.

We all went back to work.

No debriefing.

No offer of assistance.

Surprise Attack

While conducting interviews for this book, I heard hundreds of stories similar to mine. I thought one, in particular, was appropriate to add. It is a situation many have encountered, yet I have not. Therefore, I share my colleague's story.

This incident occurred in a small, critical-access emergency department. It was during a night shift, and there were only a few patients in the department. There was a patient who was very drunk and very big. The patient had been medically cleared and had gone to the bathroom. When he walked back into his room, the nurse, Brenda Little, went in with him. The patient was standing next to the gurney. He was cooperative and pleasant. Brenda was between the patient and the door to the room for safety reasons. However, she was not directly in front of the door but off to the side.

This particular little town had a high number of intoxicated individuals who frequented the ER. Because of this, there was a community detox facility. This facility was open to taking impaired patients, as long as they were able to walk.

Brenda told the patient the detox facility would take him, and he agreed to go. She told him it would be a bit of a wait before he was able to go, so she asked him if he would like some water or Gatorade. At this point, without warning, the patient lunged at Brenda. He attacked her so fast, she did not have time to scream for help. The patient grabbed her by the throat and picked her up off the ground. He then punched her in the face. Because she was not in front of the door, the other nurse could not see her. The second nurse and the tech were both small women. Even if they could see what was happening, they would have been of little help.

Brenda was eventually able to crawl out of the room. The patient exited the ER. Local police found him shortly after he left. They had to taser him twice, and then several officers were required to subdue him. He was brought back to the ER, since he had been tased, to be medically cleared. This time, it was to go to jail. Fortunately, Brenda's injuries were far less serious than they could have been. Actually, she could have been killed.

Several days after the above incident occurred, an attorney from the prosecutor's office called Brenda. He informed her his office was reducing the charges to a misdemeanor. Brenda had not even been interviewed by the prosecutor. She told him he needed to hear her story first. She recounted her horrific experience and the completely unprovoked attack. After listening to her, the prosecutor offered condolences for her experience. He then told her he was still reducing the charges because he did not want to ruin the attacker's life. Brenda protested, but to no avail. Had this person done this to a police officer, it would have been a felony and prosecuted to the full extent of the law. However, all across the country, nurses are assaulted every day, and then they just get back to work.

THE VALUE OF THERAPY

Just as it sometimes takes certain events to make us realize we are affected by what we deal with every day, it can also take a slap in the face to make us recognize the value of doing something about it, which can include some form of therapy.

It was later in my career when I would encounter an actual, effective debriefing. I was working as the medical manager (chief flight nurse) for a helicopter EMS (HEMS) operator in southern California. It was a typical Sunday evening when I received a call from my counterpart, the aviation manager, Dennis McCall. I was standing outside my house in the driveway, leaning up against my truck. Our conversation went like this:

"Hey there, D."

"Are you sitting down, Brian?"

"Should I be?"

"There is a very real possibility we just lost Air 2."

Not having any idea what he was referring to and knowing we had been short an aircraft due to scheduled maintenance, I replied:

"What now, and how long will they be out of service?"

As if he did not even hear what I said, Dennis continued:

"LifeComm (our dispatch center) and the comm center (the county EMS dispatch agency) have lost contact with Air 2, and there are multiple reports from motorists on Interstate 15 of a small aircraft crash and a fireball on the side of the hill in the Cajon Pass."

I remember sliding down against my truck, sitting on the ground, and saying:

"Oh my gosh, you are serious!"

Dennis replied to me by saying:

"This is the real deal, B. The fire department is still trying to make their way to the incident, so I don't have any more information right now."

Dennis then said:

"I need to know what medical crew members are working on Air 2 today."

I grabbed the folder containing my crew schedule. I found today's date and saw two Xs in the boxes of the duty crew for the day. I remember pausing because I did not want to run my finger across the page to the left to see what names corresponded with those Xs. I felt sick in my stomach as I told Dennis the names of the flight nurse and flight medic. I then asked him who the pilot was.

Dennis and I then had a very private and brief, yet emotional, exchange. I remember Dennis had his scanner on, and I could hear in the background, "Air 2, comm center! Air 2, comm center!" There was no reply. I then asked him, according to the PIAP (post-incident action plan) process:

"What do you need me to do?"

We had practiced our PIAP on numerous occasions, usually a chip light, or an unscheduled landing, or a myriad of other typical things that happen in the aircraft business that require an alteration in the scheduled flight plan. Dennis always insisted on going through all the steps exactly by the book so we would be well prepared if a major incident ever occurred. I admit, I often thought it was a waste of time when there was no real emergency. I had no idea how much those seemingly insignificant trips through our PIAP process were about to reveal their benefit.

Since Dennis was the first manager contacted by dispatch, he was the point person for this incident. He gave me clear instructions about who he needed me to call and what to tell them. He also reminded me not to call dispatch or anyone up the chain of command except him. I began calling flight crews at all our bases, as well as my supervisors for each base, if they were not working. It was early December, and the bustle of Christmas shopping was everywhere. I decided my very first call needed to be to Kent Sprague, my base manager of Air 2, the helicopter suspected of crashing. That call went something like this:

"Hey, Brian, how are you?"
I could hear lots of noise in the background. I replied:

"Kent, I need you to get somewhere right now where it is quiet, and we can speak without interruption." After a minute, the noise was gone. He replied:

"Sorry, my wife and I are out doing some Christmas shopping. What's up?"

I said, "It appears Air 2 has crashed."

I gave him the briefing I received from Dennis and told him we were activating our PIAP. I instructed him to call every employee from his base: pilots, medics, nurses, and mechanics. According to the PIAP, he would notify the lead pilot of his base if possible and delegate calls to him. I instructed him not to call anyone up the chain of command except for me and to instruct everyone he spoke with not to call anyone but him. I told him I would call him back with an update as soon as I had one from Dennis. He and I also had a short personal exchange, and then he did as I asked him. I placed that same call to all my other base supervisors. It was very emotional, to say the least, as I was the first person they were hearing this from, and it was shocking news.

Once I had reached everyone and relayed information and instructions to them, I called Dennis back.

"Hey, D, I have contacted everyone as you requested and was able to reach someone at each base. What now?"

After a brief pause, Dennis replied:

"The fire department has reached the crash site, B. They have confirmed it is Air 2. They requested the coroner, times three."

I had known in my heart this was what the outcome was going to be. However, hearing my friend and colleague say it to me took my breath away. After another emotional exchange, I asked for new instructions. He had a couple of logistical things for me to do. He had spoken with our program director, and we all agreed to ground our other bases for the night. However, he mostly just wanted me to update our crews. I again made phone calls to all my base supervisors with the update. I was a seasoned critical care, emergency, and flight nurse. I had already witnessed many things that would make most people's skin crawl. Nevertheless, I felt a profound sense of despair I had never experienced before in my career.

The rest of the night was filled with phone calls and making sure the family members of our deceased crew and all our employees were notified. Our PIAP system was so well rehearsed that we were able to personally contact everyone before they heard about the crash on the news. That was quite a feat, considering this was all happening during the prime time evening news cycle in southern California. Dennis's insistence on being thoroughly prepared made the process go smoothly when emotions were so high, it was difficult to think straight.

The next morning, as the sun came up, Dennis and I stood on top of a hill looking down at the crash site while the coroner removed the remains of our employees, our friends. Two days prior to the crash was our annual Christmas meeting, where all the on-duty crews flew in to be with everyone else for food and fun. As Dennis and I stood on that hill witnessing the gruesome task of the coroner, we reflected on our association with these three amazing people.

The pilot, Paul "Papi" Latour, had retired from the army. He was married to his high school sweetheart. He would frequently rub in our faces that we would never have anyone as beautiful and wonderful as his Christie. They had two wonderful children. His son, Justin, in the army like his dad, was a helicopter crew chief. They loved motorcycle riding and anything outdoors in their free time. His daughter, Christen, was the absolute apple of his eye. She was in the navy and planning a wedding. Papi was excited to walk her down the aisle.

The flight medic, Jerry Miller, was a veteran of the field. He was recently remarried and had an amazing four-year-old little girl, Molly, whose name was printed in giant letters on his flight helmet.

The flight nurse, Katrina Kish, had been working in the emergency department for years. Her husband, Tim, was a fire captain with Cal Fire. Tim and Katrina were also members of the sheriff's air search and rescue team. Katrina was finishing up her master's degree and would soon be a nurse practitioner. She also still worked shifts in the ER at Loma Linda University. She had a nine-year-old son, Stephen, who she just adored.

Dennis and I had worked with all three of them for a long time and had crewed helicopters with them all. Dennis was previously stationed at their base as the lead pilot. These were not just employees. They were our friends. Dennis had three times as many flight hours as any pilot I knew. He had flown law enforcement and spent many years training pilots and reconstructing crashes. Though he was not a medical professional by trade, he had flown EMS for years and witnessed much suffering. However, this was different. This was not just close to home. It was in the front door staring us in the face. I will be forever thankful Dennis McCall was the person standing next to me on that hill and during the entire ordeal.

The next few days were filled with plans for a memorial service and trying to make certain our crews were all solid and able to fly. We still had a very important and necessary job to do. I was told by my boss we were going to have a critical-incident debriefing at Air 2's base of operation. I remember thinking what a waste of time it would be. I had so many things to do. I wanted to be with my crew members. I was also playing a huge role in planning the memorial service. I then learned the debriefing would be led by a group of volunteers who were not even part of our company. I grumbled to Dennis and several other people. I had been in the business of life and death for over two decades, and I did not need to have some amateur psychologists trying to get into my head and see if I was okay.

On the evening of the debriefing, we gathered at the base. All the remaining Air 2 employees were there, along with our leadership team. Also present were the airport firefighters from the base, as Air 2 occupied space in the airport fire station, and the fire crews were viewed as an equal part of the Air 2 team. We were all in a huge half-circle facing a small group of strangers we had never met. I will be forever thankful for that little group of "amateur counselors."

They were members of a group called START (Surface to Air Response Team) who specialize in critical-incident stress management for air medical companies. The group's leader, Temple Fletcher, explained who they were. Each member of their team had to meet two criteria. First, they had to have worked for a HEMS company. Second, they had to have been involved with a provider during the time their company experienced a fatal incident. In other words, they had to have already walked a mile in our shoes.

Suddenly, they felt a little less like strangers. I could see in their faces the empathy they had for all of us. They knew exactly what we were going through.

The debriefing was nothing like I expected it to be. It was incredibly informal and relaxed. They started on one end of the room and simply asked, "Can you explain to the group how you heard about the crash?" This was a pretty simple question. I was the second person in the row. As I started explaining my call from Dennis, a surprising thing happened. A floodgate that was apparently holding back an enormous volume of emotions flew open, and I could barely speak. I was embarrassed. I was one of the leadership team and an experienced nurse. I was supposed to be strong for my crews. Crying in front of all these professionals was a sign of weakness, especially for a nurse.

As I struggled to tell everyone about my experience, the entire room was silent. I looked up and saw a room full of professionals in my business. Most were looking at me. None, not a single one, made me feel like I was weak or should suck it up. All I saw were the faces of compassion and empathy. It remained that way as each person took their turn explaining to us what they were doing when they received their phone call and how they responded. There were many tears and emotions.

I was completely overwhelmed. For the first time in my career, the providers were the focus of care and compassion. Those who go to work every day to do amazing things for complete strangers were finally receiving the attention I had no idea we needed. Someone actually cared about a tragedy *we* experienced. It changed something in me forever!

The debriefing I experienced after Air 2's crash, my wife's reflection of her observation in the ER, and my social media post where I tried to explain everything I had encountered over the years all helped me recognize the gross lack of attention to the providers in my business who experience relentless stressors every day at work. I began wondering what could be done about it. It was the beginning of my journey to bring much-needed awareness to this culture of neglect in my profession.

COPING

How do we cope in this business? There are several things I have done over the years, sometimes without realizing it. Many of the things in this section I have personally used as my own relief valve.

The most common coping mechanism among my colleagues is the "warped sense of humor." Some of our family and friends have seen this dark humor. Mostly, it is reserved for shoptalk. There are jokes or snide comments made, which are often, in all honesty, quite inappropriate. It is a way to separate the illness, injury, and tragedy from the victim and the family. In a sense, it is a way to dehumanize the situation so we do not see the individual(s) affected by whatever tragedy we are dealing with at that moment. I used to tell newcomers to the profession, "You need to learn to focus on the boo-boo and not the person. If you get caught up in the person, emotions can easily get in the way of critical thinking."

As I have become a more experienced nurse, I am not so sure that is the case. At least, not completely in every situation. As we get older and more experienced, our psyche develops enough callousness to allow us to let ourselves become more emotionally involved with our patients and their families. Our actions in crises become more automatic. Thus, even if we are emotionally upset by what we are encountering, we are able to continue to function in our necessary roles.

Another thing common within my profession is flirtatious conversation. Because we experience people at their most compromised, we tend to have fewer boundaries in our everyday communication with each other. Much of the time, it seems innocent. However, it often leads to another coping mechanism for some people. That is, promiscuity. In this line of work, I believe, more so than in others, affairs are quite common. Of course, this is reflected in the high divorce rate within the field. It is one of the many destructive activities engaged in.

Drinking is another popular pastime. It continues to amaze me how many married or otherwise committed individuals will go out with a group of colleagues after work for drinks and food, instead of going straight home to their families. Night-shifters do this as often as the day crew; they just go out drinking in the morning. It is an opportunity to humanize each other. I have friends tell me they like seeing each other outside of the work environment and being able to spend time with people who can relate to them.

For me, reaching out to my family was one way to cope. There were times, as a young ER nurse, when I would encounter a child—the same age as one of my own children—who would die, and I watched parents grieve. I remember working the night shift and calling home after such incidents. I would wake my wife and ask her to check on the children and make sure they were okay. She did not ask me what happened. She knew I was not telling her for a reason. I usually could not tell her. Mostly because if I tried to tell her at that moment, I would likely just cry. I asked her to give them a kiss for me. I would wait on the phone, and she would come back and assure me they were all okay and that she had kissed them and whispered in their ear, "Daddy loves you." She knew I would probably tell her about it when I got home and was ready and able to talk about it.

Getting together with colleagues is another great way to debrief. After the experience of losing three friends in the helicopter crash and the subsequent debriefing, I did not talk much about the incident or my feelings. Many months after the crash, we were over at my friend Dennis's home for a visit. I remember we were sitting in his Jacuzzi with our wives. The ladies went to get something, and Dennis and I began to talk about the night he called to tell me about the crash. Later, the girls told us they could hear our conversation and left us alone.

Dennis and I had a very personal conversation about what we were doing and thinking the night the crash's aftermath unfolded. I did not realize at the time what great therapy that was for both of us. Up to that point, I had never really had a discussion with a colleague about anything stressful from work. Perhaps it was because Dennis is also my very good friend, and I felt comfortable talking to him. I think it also may have something to do with the fact he is not a medical person, and it was not a threat to my ego to have him see my emotions when I spoke of the crash. Unfortunately, though we shared a bit of our feelings with each other, we did not express how deeply affected we each really were. Regardless, I was glad to have the discussion.

Being able to discuss our emotions and be honest and vulnerable with someone may be one of the best ways to cope. Of course, as I have stated, this is likely the most difficult of all. Eighteen years after the crash, while wrapping up the writing of this book, I had a long conversation with Dennis. Though we have stayed in touch via social media and text messaging, we had not actually spoken for over a decade. As we spoke, I asked him about his career and why he was no longer flying. Understand, this man LOVED to fly. He was my absolute favorite pilot. Not only had we been part of the leadership team together, but we had also flown scores of missions together. When Dennis did his first ride-along flight with our company, it was my very first mission as a new flight nurse, just off of orientation. We literally grew up in HEMS together.

I wondered why he stopped, so I asked him. He answered me with two words: "The crash." We then spent a long time on the phone and opened up to each other. I shared with him the amount of stress I felt during the time of the crash. It had taken an enormous toll on me. I had trouble sleeping and became detached from the people closest to me. At the time, I admired Dennis because he seemed so stoic. He was a rock during the crash's aftermath. He had gone on to become the director of operations and chief pilot for the entire corporation after I left the company. It was a job he was immensely qualified for. I assumed he moved up because that was a natural path for him. Dennis shared how profoundly stressed the entire ordeal made him. He told me the reason he went into upper management was to get away from the cockpit and to distance himself from the crash.

I was stunned. I had no idea how much he was emotionally suffering from the crash. Dennis said he thought I was a rock during the crash's aftermath and let it just roll off my shoulders. He, too, was stunned to realize how difficult a time I had had. We each assumed the other was perfectly okay. How terribly wrong we were. It is so ironic that the very person I could have, and should have, talked to about what I felt then had been feeling the same way I had.

In our phone call, we shared with each other our individual experiences with therapy and trying to deal with the emotional trauma we endured. Dennis had gone on to be the point person for thirteen more crashes the corporation had across the country. Though he was doing a job he was born for, it was the exposure to more crash aftermaths that greatly contributed to his leaving the business altogether. Our conversation allowed us to rekindle a line of communication that we both vowed to never let go silent again.

E FOR EFFORT

The details of traumatic cases spread throughout the department, which nearly always happens in the ER. As I was working on this book, I accepted my first travel assignment. It was in the emergency department of a major Level 1 trauma center. This particular facility did not assign travelers as primary nurses to traumas, regardless of one's experience. I think this is good practice, since the knowledge of the specific department and process is more important in a chaotic situation. For me, that was a blessing, as I was at a point in my career where I was comfortable doing whatever I needed to do and would rather not do more.

On this particular day, I was in the room of one of my patients, starting an IV and drawing labs. I heard a page in the ER: "Critical trauma in the RS (receiving suite) now." I was a bit surprised because there is usually an overhead page letting the staff know something like this is coming, as well as the ETA. I assumed I had missed the first page. There are nurses assigned to trauma and plenty of young, hungry nurses willing to go help, so I continued what I was doing.

Let's return to the present ER, while I was talking to "central." I could see almost every nurse headed over to the trauma suites, and it was automatic for me to just stay back. Of course, in short order, the nurses who were not needed in the trauma rooms came back to the floor.

Eventually, we all became aware of the details surrounding this incident. There was a small family of three. A young couple and their eighteen-month-old child. The father was in the military and on a training assignment across the country. The mother was lonely, and one of her cousins was flying out to spend time with her and her child. A friend was taking the mom and baby to the airport, and traffic slowed to a stop on the freeway. While stopped, their car died. After a short time, traffic began to move; however, they could not get the car started. Without warning, a full-sized pickup slammed into the back of this tiny car at 70 mph. The mother and toddler were in the back seat and were pushed up into the front seat. The accident was devastating.

Immediately, a basic life support (BLS) transfer ambulance— which is responsible for transferring relatively stable patients between hospitals and from nursing homes to appointments— came upon the accident. This crew was very young and had almost no experience with 911 calls, least of all the kind of disastrous crash they were about to encounter. The EMTs were flagged down, so they stopped and entered the scene. What they found was horrific. The mother and toddler were severely injured and completely unconscious.

This nonemergency crew made a split-second decision that was exactly the correct one. They realized it would take at least ten minutes for paramedics to arrive on scene. They were on the freeway, just three minutes away from the top trauma center in the state—ours. They decided to load the mom and toddler into their ambulance and drive like mad to our facility while trying to do what they could. The drivers of the car and truck were "walking wounded." They were not critical, so this BLS crew raced to our ER with this mom and toddler. They detected no signs of life from either and started CPR on the toddler. Since they are not a 911 crew, they had no way of notifying our facility that they were on the way. Our trauma teams had absolutely no time to prepare. The crew pulled into the ambulance bay and backed in. Fortunately, there were local city paramedic units parked in the ambulance bay, cleaning their rigs. The BLS driver jumped out and alerted the paramedic units to what they had and asked for help. The medics rushed to help, grabbed the child, and brought him in first.

When they entered the ER, our staff was completely surprised by their presence. This is when the first call went out that a "critical trauma" was here. Right behind the child was the mother, thus the second call. We were an academic facility with a residency program in the ER. This means there were two attending ER physicians and several ER resident physicians at various levels of training. There was also an army of experienced nurses and techs. What happened in that moment was awesome. The staff jumped in and went to work.

For those reading this who work in busy trauma centers, this is not a surprise. When you do this level of trauma so often, most of what is done is so repetitive, it is automatic. Muscle memory, if you will. The child had devastating injuries, and after only a relatively short resuscitation attempt, he was pronounced dead. The mother's injuries were not so obvious, and she was worked on longer. However, it was quickly apparent her injuries were fatal, and she, too, was pronounced dead.

The two attending physicians reached out to the military. They had a video chat with the husband and father. He was on the other end of the video with a commanding officer and a military chaplain.

The ER physicians, via video, explained to this young man that in the blink of an eye, his little family had been wiped out.

The fire department did respond to the scene, and the driver of the car was brought to our emergency department as well. He was in a room close to me. I could hear the staff saying he had no idea the condition of his friends. The news of the accident spread like wildfire, and a somber atmosphere was noticeable in the entire department. This is how it goes.

Those close to the patients are obviously affected. What we tend to forget are those who were not in the room. They are affected as well. Partly because of the story of what happened with regard to the accident, but also the knowledge that this little family was changed in the blink of an eye, and it happened, or was finalized, in our midst. It brings a real sense of our own mortality to light and the realization that, as in the proverbial saying, "There, but for the grace of God, go I." This could have been any one of us or our family. This is another source of stress in our world. At various steps along the way in one's career, there are close friends and family members who are of the same age as those who experience tragedy in our midst. For me, as previously mentioned, it was when my children were young. It is difficult not to wonder how devastating the anguish of the surviving family members is when, "It could just as easily have been me."

In most of the preceding examples, it ended with the fact that we all went back to work without anyone checking on us. This time, it was different. Later in the day, another page was made in the ER: "Attention staff, there will be a debriefing in the trauma room beginning immediately." I had not been present in the crisis. I was also a new traveler, and hardly anyone in the department knew who I was. However, I felt compelled to attend this debriefing. Mostly for research sake, as I had the opportunity to be present when a debrief was being held in a major trauma center very shortly after a devastatingly traumatic incident occurred. There was no way I could pass up the opportunity to get some real-time research for this book. My patients were all chill, so I went to the trauma suite. I snuck in and went into the radiology control room off to the side, where nobody could see me but where I could hear everything being said. I got out a piece of paper and waited.

I must emphasize something here. What I am going to point out about my observations is not meant to be viewed as negative toward anyone present in the debrief. In fact, there were several things I was profoundly impressed with and will mention. Nobody present had formal training on how to conduct such a debrief. Those who organized it were aware enough to realize the gravity of the situation and how it was necessary to talk about it and check on the staff. I applaud the attending physician for taking the initiative to organize this debrief, knowing the effect it had on the entire department. In my forty years doing this business, I can count on one hand the number of times this has happened. This doctor is a rock star in my eyes.

Some of the first comments made by one of the physicians gave me pause. It was not what he said, but how I could tell it was received, based on the looks some of the staff had. When he made his comments, there was no doubt in my mind his intentions were pure. He was doing his best to help those in the room keep things in perspective. The look on the faces of the staff present was mostly despair. The comment made was, "Remember, this is not about us." I assumed he was trying to remind everyone not to personalize the situation. However, the comment was made after outlining the debrief and what we were there to accomplish, which was to answer any questions the staff had about what was done and the decisions in both cases to cease resuscitative efforts.

My first thought was, "This, the debrief, IS about us. In fact, it is only about us." I assume he was speaking about the trauma, but it seemed like he was talking about the debriefing. In spite of great intentions, we often make our colleagues feel like they need to suck it up and move on. Though not his intention, it is how it was received by some staff.

Another comment from someone else in the room was, "These things happen. It is just the way it is." Everyone in this line of work understands these things happen. That is, the human side of the staff. Even though we know what might come through the doors during our shift, we are still human and have real feelings. Debriefings should focus on the staff and the real possibility there are some in the room struggling. When we give the impression this stuff is just part of the job and we are supposed to suck it up, those who are suffering will rarely reach out for help. This is feeding the culture of "We just don't talk about it."

The takeaway from this debriefing was, still, mostly positive. A very aware doctor knew the emotional toll this type of incident has on people. What I wish is that there would be formal training in hospitals for these types of debriefs so words are chosen more carefully. If there were an effective training program in this hospital, there is no doubt the doctor who organized this debrief, would be eager to attend.

As I already described, my flight program had a fatal crash. I outlined my communications with Dennis and how we recently opened up to each other about what we experienced emotionally.

More recently, I reached out to one of my former flight medics, Jake Warner. He had made a post on social media a while back, indicating he had residual stress after the crash. He was one of my best medics. I had interviewed and hired him. He loved flying and performed brilliantly in the high-intensity world of flight medicine. He eventually left patient care for a career in medical devices. I asked him to tell me his story. As with Dennis, he focused on "the crash" and how he was emotionally injured following the accident.

As Jake and I talked, I realized something very profound. I have interviewed hundreds of people for this book. I racked my brain by trying to think of who I would talk to regarding stress in this business. While talking with Jake, I realized I had never, even one time, thought about talking to a single one of my flight crews up until that point. It is as if I had blocked that event out and, in so doing, blocked out all my amazing crew members. As Jake recounted the struggles he had been through since the crash, I felt sick that I had never had a debriefing for my crews.

Of course, I did not have the knowledge I do now regarding moral injury and traumatic stress. Still, I could not help but feel terrible for not doing something for my crews. It made me profoundly aware I was in the exact cultural mindset as the hospital administration from the story of the young woman who shot herself. That is, it was not a priority to explore more deeply the possibility of moral injury to my crews and to offer them real assistance. Even after the debriefing we had for the Air 2 crew members and our leadership team, I never thought to organize something for my own people. I knew it helped me. I knew it was a positive process. Yet because of the culture, I did not think this was something that would be universally beneficial to all the employees of my flight program.

At the end of my discussion with Jake, I asked him a question. "If I had organized a debriefing like the one I attended for you guys, do you think you would still be flying?" Jake took a minute and then said, "Yes, I think I would." This hit me like a ton of bricks. I had asked all my crews if they were okay. But I now know that was not nearly enough.

Silent Trauma: The side of healthcare we don't talk about

Reflecting back on my own ignorance of the profundity of what we do makes me more determined to do what I can to change the culture.

CHANGING THE CULTURE

"A person's countenance does not always reflect what they are really thinking. They may not be okay!"

Mary Wagner, RN

Emergency Services

Ronald Reagan UCLA Medical Center, July 5, 2021

In order to change anything, we must first recognize there is a problem and then begin to look for a source. Just knowing there is a problem is not enough. If I come home and my basement is flooded, I know there is a problem. However, I cannot fix the problem until I know the source. The water might be coming from a broken pipe in the house. Maybe a sink or toilet or shower. Perhaps it is the main water line coming into the house. It could be a leak outside, flooding the window well and seeping in through it. The flood is not actually the problem. It is the consequence of whatever the main problem is, which is the leak in this example. In order to stop the problem and effectively deal with the consequences, the problem must be identified. The same applies to the toxic culture in emergency services. There are many sources where stressors come from. However, what I believe is the most profound problem will not win me any popularity contests with my colleagues.

I believe we, the emergency services workers, are our own worst enemy when it comes to the toxic culture. We tolerate, we adapt, we improvise, we ignore, we go with the flow, and we are afraid to speak out or speak up. We are quick to complain to each other but afraid to take corrective action. Part of this is an environment of fearing for our jobs. Part of it is not wanting to look weak to our colleagues. Ironically, griping and complaining without offering a solution through the proper channels is, in my opinion, a sign of true weakness. It takes courage to stand up to those in leadership, especially if they are managers more than they are leaders.

As I began looking for material written about this topic, I discovered a couple of things. First, there were no books about this specific topic regarding nursing I could find. I found several articles and periodicals that had been penned over the years. The vast majority were written by doctors about doctors, specifically resident physicians. Many of these articles were about emergency services, and most were about the stress of long hours worked.

Much has been written about combat stress. There is quite a movement to recognize the stressors of first responders and law enforcement. I did discover a common conclusion, which was quite disturbing, though not surprising. With virtually no exception, each of the articles written about the effects of stress inside and out of the hospital had a common finding.

After making the case of stress affecting those who work in this business, the authors all made a similar observation. That is, we all know these jobs are stressful; however, in this business, *we just don't talk about it*. Let that sink in for a minute. We don't talk about it? How can that be? We are in the business of trying to figure out what is bothering people so we can help them. That includes physical, emotional, and mental help. How, then, did *we* ever allow a culture to develop where we keep our own mental health hush-hush? We tell other people who are the primary caregivers of patients to take care of themselves, or they will be no good to anyone. This applies to parents, spouses, children who care for elderly parents, and paid personal caregivers. Yet somehow, this advice is never directed back at us. This should especially apply to those of *us* whose profession it is to care for people.

Silent Trauma: The side of healthcare we don't talk about

The key takeaway to what I just stated is, how did WE ever allow a culture like this to develop? The answer is we are born, metaphorically, into it and relearn it every day. Then, we become very good at recognizing it and complaining to all our colleagues about it. Finally, and tragically, we then perpetuate it onto our professional offspring, and the cycle goes on and on and on!

ER staff, like first responders, do not get the benefit of screening who we care for. We are obligated to take care of whoever is put before us and under whatever circumstances put them there. Because of this, we tend to view ourselves as the best of the best. I am not saying we *are* the best. I am simply pointing out what we think. We, by the nature of the job, can handle anything. We must. Were it not so, we could not do what we do effectively. However, "can handle anything" needs to be defined. In the emergency room specifically, we can be completely overwhelmed, just like every other area of healthcare. However, there is a unique difference.

Let's look at what can happen on any given day, hypothetically. Imagine we are in the ER. The department is full, and there are a large number of people in the waiting room. We are a major trauma center with a full complement of resources. We are cruising along and getting things done. (Let's use one of my former hospital demographics, specifically. We have fifty-four treatment beds, eight of them designated for trauma. At capacity, we have five attending physicians and a full staff of twenty-five nurses and seven techs.) All our rooms are full. We have a few other receiving hospitals in the area. We have several critical-care level patients: septic shock, respiratory failure, diabetic ketoacidosis, etc. We are stretched a little thin, but it's not something we are not prepared for. We have five ambulances waiting for a bed to offload their patients. We then get two ambulance calls of patients coming in. One is a heart attack (STEMI, for my clinical peeps) and the other is an acute stroke.

Now we are a bit on edge. Each of these patients will require immediate attention and additional staff. We decide to close the ER to ambulance traffic and go on "diversion." This means no ambulances can come to us unless the patient is in extremis, meaning life-or-death. Before either of the two critical patients arrives, we get a call about an MCI (multi-casualty incident), with four trauma patients coming to us. We are a trauma center and cannot say no, even though we are closed to regular ambulance traffic. Now we are in crisis mode. The charge nurse notifies up the food chain and gets permission to close the ER due to an internal disaster. We are completely maxed out and cannot take another patient, especially a really sick one. Everyone is working at maximum capacity. We have additional staff from other departments, but we are still crazy busy. At least we are closed for everything and will be able to get on top of things before opening back up again. Well, not so fast.

A frantic parent comes running in the front door with a child who is barely breathing and blue. Right beyond her is a middle-aged man who is profusely sweating and complaining of crushing chest pressure. What I just described actually happens. Many will say it is an extreme example, and they would be correct. However, it is an extreme example of what happens on a smaller scale every day in ERs all over the world. That is, no matter how busy you think you are and how much you do to mitigate the circumstances, you cannot ever close the doors completely. The last two patients I described are here. You have no staff. Absolutely no resources to deal with them. However, you must deal with them and do it quickly and efficiently. Their lives depend on it.

We have several patients in this scenario who are ready to go upstairs to the ICU, but the department is full and has no beds for them. So we deal with them. We have no other choice. Staff are maxed out and stressed because they are trying to figure out how to prioritize many critically ill patients. Many staff are emotionally overwhelmed and need to walk away and collect their thoughts. However, human nature and their sense of clinical responsibility prevent them from doing it. They are compelled to stay in the fight because lives, literally, depend on it.

The above scenario is an explanation of the uniqueness of the emergency room. Every other department in the hospital can be too full to accept another patient. Only the ER cannot do this. The other exception is labor and delivery triage for those hospitals with this service. Some would say EMS is the same. Generally speaking, it is not. I have worked in EMS for years. Most of the time, there are not so many calls backed up so you never get a break. In many cases, EMS has bases of operations where they post and wait for a call to be dispatched. My message in this book does apply to EMS and law enforcement and everyone who deals with human tragedy on a regular basis. All who work in emergency services, in and out of a hospital setting, have a unique situation within the profession.

The reason we, in emergency services, have the mindset of being able to deal with "anything" is because we have to in order to be able to do our jobs. Yes, we can handle anything, with respect to getting the job done in the moment. That is what we are really talking about. It does not mean we can handle anything emotionally. At least, not always alone. I am trying to bring to light there is a difference, and we must stop conflating the two.

The culture of keeping a stiff upper lip and pretending to those around us we are not bothered by what we see is madness. Yet that is exactly what we do. As new members of the team in emergency services, you first encounter trainers or preceptors. These experienced workers have learned to keep their emotions at bay. They must project confidence and grit to the new people. They must show they are decisive and stoic when faced with tragedy. The culture dictates there is no way they can show their emotional response to a crisis while training someone else. To do so would show weakness.

On the flip side, they must also project that same persona to their manager, lest they be seen as someone too weak to coach new employees. The new person rarely, if ever, sees an experienced colleague emotionally upset by what they are experiencing. Instead, the seasoned staff will often make inappropriate jokes in the middle of the tragedy. This projects to the new employee that seasoned employees are not affected by this type of thing. In fact, they are able to make jokes about it. Thus, the cycle is passed on to the new person. They learn, by observing, how they are "supposed" to behave in crises. If they are emotionally touched, and they most certainly are, they had better not let it show. What they do not realize is many of the things they see senior personnel doing are coping mechanisms to deal with the stress. Ironically, the inappropriate jokes, sarcasm, and other responses appear to some as signs the trauma is not affecting these people, when they are actually tools being used to deal with or mask the stress they experience.

Let me be clear. I am not suggesting we are doing anything wrong by pushing through emotional turmoil and getting the job done. As I have repeatedly stated, we need to be able to get the job done in the moment, and this is also something we need to teach new people to be able to do. We are in a profession where we have chosen to do hard things during very traumatic situations. Many times, others' lives depend on us doing what is necessary without hesitation. If we cannot work through our own emotions, regardless of their profundity, we may cause great harm to another human being. The people we care for come to us specifically because they expect us to be able to help them. This creates a dichotomy.

So how do we change the culture in emergency services? In part, we have to look at ourselves and understand we are *all* affected. As with people engaging in addictive behavior, recognition is the first step. As a profession, we must admit there is a problem. If the profession as a whole does not recognize this, it is a waste of time going any further.

In healthcare, there is no shortage of continuing education available. There are classes provided by hospitals, on the internet, professional organizations, conferences, and a myriad of other venues to promote education. Of the seemingly countless topics covered in continuing education venues, there are virtually no courses offered regarding the kind of stress I am speaking of. This is due to the fact there is no real category for the subject matter. The closest thing at the time of writing of this book is probably "productive work environment." There is rarely anything about traumatic stress. Nursing and other healthcare organizations must get on board and request speakers who can address this topic frequently. At conferences, there are classes on new medical techniques, care plans, equipment, social justice topics, workplace violence, recognizing abused children, recognizing stress in our patients (a little irony there), career advancement, advanced certifications, and many other topics. But this topic is usually found in a breakout session mixed in with everything else. It needs to be a prevailing theme at these venues. It needs to be a keynote address to the body of the conference.

Once the profession begins to take it seriously and make it a major topic of importance, it will be infinitely easier to openly discuss and address it. I recently spoke at the National Emergency Nurses Association Conference. This conference was attended by thousands of ER nurses. The very hardened "we can do anything" crowd I am writing about. There were many great topics and sessions I attended, and three of the sessions were packed: "Nurse Burnout," "It's Okay to Say I Am Not Okay," and "Traumatic Stress." The first two were in large rooms. However, they were full, and not everyone who wanted in could attend. The third was the session I presented. It was in the exhibit hall, so there was no restriction keeping people from standing in the back. Why were these three sessions so wildly popular? Because we *are* all affected by what we experience, and we know it!

Nurses with the most experience are a key factor. For the most part, in every profession, new people look up to the staff with the most longevity. Therefore, those with the most seniority need to be involved in recognizing the importance of detoxing emotionally. Part of the orientation process into the emergency environment must include discussions about traumatic stress. In fact, this discussion should begin in nursing and medical schools, paramedic programs, and organizational orientations.

Hospitals need to be involved as well. If they have an initiative to address the mental health of their staff, especially in the emergency department, it will become infinitely easier to bring awareness to the staff. There also needs to be processes in place to address the stress experienced by their staff. When a major incident occurs, it is easy to select the employees involved in that particular incident and organize a debriefing for them, even though this is rarely done. However, recognizing the signs of stress and helping the employees who are affected by the cumulative stressors is not as easy. I am referring to the day-to-day grind of relentless crises emergency workers face. A system must be put in place to check the emotional pulse of all staff members on a regular basis, in real time, to see where they are. There must be a process where a post-incident checkup can be done immediately following an event, when the staff involved are expected to continue with their shift. As Zig Ziglar always said, we need a regular "checkup from the neck up (Ziglar)." It is important to understand who was affected and to what degree. Most staff will be able to get back in the game right away. Some will not be able to, depending on their involvement in the event and where they are in their life, career, and current emotional state.

Some staff will reach a breaking point due to a seemingly insignificant event because it is the final contributor that causes their cumulative stress tank to overflow. Often, when this happens, other staff are scratching their heads and assume their colleague must have something going on at home because there is nothing at work that should have caused a reasonable person to be upset. These are some of the most important situations to look for. We have been conditioned to expect some people to show emotions during major incidents. However, the nature of emergency services is repetitive and constant chaos. Therefore, we tune out most things around us. Just like when my wife was with me in the ER and I did not notice any of the things she was keenly aware of, we tune out the majority of things going on in the ER every day, especially if we are not directly involved. The breaking point incident for some may be unnoticed by everyone else. It may be something as simple as a child crying and looking to a parent when the lab tech is in the room drawing blood. This is something that may happen many times in a shift. However, seeing the anguish on that small child's face may be the final incident after years of stressors that put a particular person over the edge. Understanding how cumulative stress is equally or more profound than one major tragedy is crucial in understanding traumatic stress and beginning to break the culture of dismissing it.

By the nature of what we do, it is impossible to close for an hour or two so the staff can regroup. Being able to evaluate staff and give them a quick mental checkup is not so simple when the flood of patients keeps coming. However, it is important to make certain the staff are mentally able to press forward. Even staff who appear to be okay may be struggling. In this business, it is imperative for those performing critical interventions to completely have their head in the game.

Virtually every healthcare organization has an employee assistance program (EAP) in place. This usually consists of the employee being able to have three visits with a counselor of some sort as part of their benefits package. This could be for marriage, family, or personal counseling. It is confidential, and the employer has no idea what the employee is seeking assistance for. Though this is a good start, it is a far cry from what is actually needed. First, in most cases, it will take three sessions just to get the emergency services employee to open up and speak freely about what they are dealing with, assuming they are willing to talk to someone at all. Second, there needs to be professionals available who specialize in emergency services staff. That is, counselors who are trained to work with employees in emergency services and who have specific training in getting staff to open up. They need to understand this specific patient population.

My personal opinion throughout the majority of my career regarding therapists was pretty jaded. It goes something like this:

I am a nurse. I am nationally certified in critical care, emergency, and flight nursing. I deal with traumatic cases every day. I have seen enough trauma to make most therapists need their own therapy. I am the guy who helps people who cannot deal with their stress, not the guy who needs someone to help me. Therapists are the people who get paid to help their clients make excuses for bad behavior. They are quacks. They think they know so much about how everyone else thinks and why, just because they had some classes about it and read some books. Therapists hear about tragedy from their clients, but most have never experienced the type we see every day. How in the world can someone who experiences traumatic stress vicariously through other people ever think they have any idea what is in my head? They expect me to sit down and have a feel-good, kumbaya visit with them so they can listen to me and ask, "How does that make you feel?" In my profession, we often laugh about people who go to therapy because they cannot deal with the real world and need someone else to hold their hand.

Before you start defending therapists, if you have taken offense at what you just read, remember something. What I just shared as my historical view of therapists is what most in emergency services believe. At the very least, we believe no general therapist has an idea how many tragedies are jammed into our heads after years of repetitive exposure. That is exactly what I thought about therapists for most of my career, and I must admit, I still feel this way. This illustrates what a significant portion of emergency services employees think as well, regardless of the reality. But, I am the guy who the therapist is going to meet. I am the guy who has no idea how much he may actually need the therapist. The therapist I go to must understand who I am and what my experiences are. They need to have a real understanding of what it is like to deal with the types of traumatic stress I have experienced over and over. More importantly, they need to understand how profoundly difficult it is for me to share my experiences, the deep emotional part of them, with someone who has not been there. Hospitals need to have a network of therapists who understand this. They need to be specialized in interacting with me, a guy who has built up a fifty-foot wall around myself to keep therapists out.

Hospitals and organizations in the business of emergency services need to first understand there is a problem in their midst with traumatic stress. Then they need to make certain there are specific therapists in place for employees to go to, but finding the appropriate therapists who specialize in emergency services workers is a real problem. When entertaining the idea of writing this book, I was directed to exactly the type of therapist we need. Her name is Tania Glenn. She began her road to becoming a social worker without a clear vision of who her clientele would be or where her practice would lead her. Toward the end of her training, she was drawn to working with first responders. Then, just after she finished her training and was considering how to proceed with her practice, the bombing of the federal building in Oklahoma City happened. She went to the scene to see if she could be of help. She was assigned to work with first responders. This is where the love affair began.

Tania has spent the entirety of her career working with first responders, law enforcement, flight crews, emergency services workers, and the military. She has logged more ride-along hours and shadowing of staff than most full-time employees in the business have with only a few years under their belt. Tania is not a medical clinician. She does not do the job we do. However, she has immersed herself in what we do so she can understand exactly what the clientele she loves so much are going through. She understands, better than anyone else in her field, how those in my profession view those in her profession. She gets our skepticism and how tightly closed our ranks are to prevent outsiders from entering our circle. She knows we are a different breed and require a unique approach if we are going to open up to an outsider, especially a therapist.

Because she specializes in what we do, she is not overwhelmed by the stories she hears from us. I am not saying she is not affected. I am certain she is. However, she is not shocked. She is able to listen as a colleague would and use her clinical expertise to intervene and treat her clients. She is not the only therapist out there who understands us. However, she is one of the very few who specialize in us. She, along with those who share her expertise, is precisely who we need to be directed to when we reach out for help. In my opinion, she is the leading expert on treating traumatic stress and moral injury in emergency services workers. I know, because I have been in her office as a client. Anyone reading this who thinks they need to speak with someone who gets it, reach out to her. (Tania Glenn & Associates, PA.)

One of the speakers I met at a recent Emergency Nurses Association Conference, Brandi Beers, shared her story with me. She is an experienced ER nurse who went into flight nursing. She loves being a nurse and loves flight nursing. She has seen many stressful things in her career. While flying, she responded to a particularly traumatic call. It was traumatic physically for the patient and emotionally for all involved. In Brandi's words, she felt like she made life-saving decisions in the moment, and then questioned if it was the correct thing to do after the fact. In the days following the incident, she really struggled with what she had experienced.

This incident was the straw that broke her camel's back. After years of traumatic events, her moral tank finally overflowed. Brandi has a sweet nature and is generally kind, but she became curt and was difficult to work with, according to her. She requested a session with a therapist through her company's EAP. When she met with this therapist and began sharing her experiences in graphic detail, the therapist vomited in the trash can. This was likely an experienced therapist. I am sure she was trained and qualified in general practice. Her intentions were good, and she wanted to help Brandi. However, she was completely ill-equipped to deal with the profoundly traumatic experiences this flight nurse was laying out. Here is a nurse who is reaching out for help. She goes through the proper channels and utilizes the well-meaning resources of her employer. Yet by the end of her first session, the therapist needed a therapist.

Fortunately, Brandi found Tania Glenn and was able to work through her challenges. She is thriving and continues to fly and speak to nursing groups. Incidentally, Brandi's presentation at the conference was titled, "It's Okay to Say I'm Not Okay."

This is representative of the majority of therapists. Not the visceral response this therapist had. Rather, the fact that most therapists have not experienced the level of traumatic events those of us working in emergency services have encountered. It is important for the hospitals, as well as EMS agencies and providers, to provide resources specifically trained and qualified to deal with the experiences emergency service workers need to share.

WHAT CAN WE DO?

I have covered many types of stressors and used real examples to highlight their emotional impact. Understanding just how many types of stressors exist, professionally, in our line of work, can seem overwhelming. Realizing we are all affected to some degree by these stressors positions us to be able to act on our own behalf and that of others. The culture within emergency services of "suck it up and move on" makes it difficult to see the personal side of how a support system helps people, in general, process tragedy in a way that helps reduce the negative effects.

I worked with an EMT named Darien Williams, who shared his very personal story with me. Darien was born as an identical twin. His mother struggled with her weight and had several other health issues, including a seizure disorder. When he was just two years old, his father committed suicide. As an adult, Darien has no memory of his father. His mother became his total foundation in life.

Silent Trauma: The side of healthcare we don't talk about

When he and his brother were five years old, their mother was sitting in her wheelchair and had a seizure. He and his brother had seen this before, so it was not particularly traumatic. However, his mother slumped down in her wheelchair, and her neck rested on the side rail of a portable toilet she was trying to get on when the seizure began. Her breathing became noisy and strange due to the side rail obstructing her airway.

Darien and his brother could tell she was in trouble and frantically tried to lift their mother off the side rail of the wheelchair to clear her airway from being occluded. In spite of their best efforts, they were unable to move her, and she stopped breathing. By the time help arrived, it was too late, and she died.

As I heard this story, I tried to remember when I was five. I cannot imagine the guilt and emotional trauma these two little boys felt. Darien's grandmother stepped in. She moved into the house and took over raising the boys. Their mother had been very active in a local church. Darien told me he remembered his mother telling him to remain active in the church if anything ever happened to her. Fortunately, the boys continued attending with their grandmother. Darien told me the familiarity of people from the church and the support they received was a lifesaver.

Just when these two boys seemed to have stability back in their lives, their grandmother got sick with cancer and passed away. They were placed in foster care for a short time. Eventually, an uncle was able to secure guardianship and adopt them. Thankfully, during the ordeal, the boys remained together.

Darien struggled during his teenage years and suffered from the trauma of the event with his mother; however, he said having a support system made all the difference in helping him eventually process what he had been through. Darien is now a veteran of the United States military and is working toward becoming a firefighter.

Sometimes, it is easier to see the traumatic stress effects on an individual when it is not related to our profession. As with Darien, many people have traumas in life that affect them deeply. When we look at an individual's personal trials, it is easy for us to see the trauma they have faced and know they need support. This is something we do every day in our careers. Why, then, is it so difficult for us to realize the trauma we are faced with in dealing with other people's tragedies is a real thing?

Silent Trauma: The side of healthcare we don't talk about

It is the same with our complete understanding that our patients and their families need support. We ask if they would like us to call someone. We call our social workers. We do this because having support seems intuitive. Yet it seems so hard to see it as caregivers. Of course, if we have a support system, we will be better able to handle and process the accumulation of traumatic events we encounter in our profession. However, we tend to think just being there is effective support for our colleagues. Sometimes, perhaps many times, it is enough, but without understanding how deeply our colleagues may be affected at any given point, we cannot effectively support them.

I have tried to illustrate how dismissive the culture of emergency services tends to be of care providers who have experienced stress through a single event or an accumulation of events. This has nothing to do with a lack of empathy on our part. It is because the culture we exist in does not allow us time to stop and check on those who are busy checking on everyone else. Also, since the culture tells us we are not allowed to be affected, perhaps, subconsciously, we assume all our colleagues are good to go.

Why, then, write this book? Because illustrating the types of stressors we face is important. However, breaking the culture of sucking it up is the primary reason. In order to do this, we need to be actively involved in caring for ourselves and each other as much as we do for our patients and their families. Creating an environment where it is not awkward to check on each other's mental health depends on all of us buying into the belief that, "It is okay to say I am not okay." Though being willing to step up and be proactive is not necessarily enough if we do not have the proper training and support to deal with traumatic issues.

We all need to take basic steps when we feel overwhelmed, emotionally. Remember, this may not happen during or immediately after a major event. It may not even happen at work. Small events during patient interaction or even at home can be the final straw, or trigger, that opens your full emotional tank. It may even surprise you how overcome with emotions you are. Recognize it for what it is. Start by reaching out to a trusted colleague or supervisor. If you feel more resources are needed, move up the chain of command. Whatever is decided, do not sit idly by waiting for someone else to act. Nursing is the largest population of employees in every medical setting. There are many online nurse content creators who provide a voice for nursing staff. Reach out to them. Join their groups. See what others are doing and ask them questions about how they seek assistance in their respective organizations. Someone needs to take the first step. Why not you?

WHAT IF

Since I began writing this book seven years ago, much has changed. Initially, I could not find anything on the subject. Now there are hundreds of articles and a handful of studies written about traumatic stress. I have reviewed a couple of dozen for publication, yet the conclusion of every paper is something like, "Yes, there is stress. We need more studies." However, little has been done. Conference planners still seem to value every other topic over this one. I have submitted to speak at a dozen conferences and am often rejected because there are too many submissions on other topics.

What if every organization put a specially trained peer support group in place?

What if every nursing school, paramedic program, EMT course, and medical school integrated this subject into their curriculum?

What if every hospital, fire department, EMS provider, and law enforcement agency included this subject in their orientation and training programs?

What if every community had specially trained therapists who specialize in emergency services employees?

What if every conference organizer included this topic as a necessity in their lineup and used speakers on this subject for their keynote addresses?

What if the moral and psychological health of emergency services employees were equally important as clinical and operational skills when continuing education programs were designed?

What if every employee looked out for their colleagues and recognized early signs of stress and PTSD?

I think we would have staff in the workforce who are as mentally healthy as they are physically. We would have fewer people leaving the profession early. This would make for a more mature workforce with a higher level of collective experience in each department. Longevity and more experienced staff improve confidence and reduce anxiety. A happier, more confident workforce has a positive impact on productivity. In healthcare, this means better patient outcomes and higher satisfaction. Higher patient satisfaction equals happier leadership. Happier leadership should lead to more resources being poured into what makes the difference.

Employees will be valued, and our mental health will be recognized. This, in turn, makes us more productive. Ultimately, we will find more joy in our work and, in turn, our lives. As we continue to encounter traumatic stress, we will have the tools and resources to cope. More importantly, the culture will have changed, and we will find it infinitely easier to reach out for help when we need it, without fear of what others may think.

I call on all those working in emergency services and healthcare as a whole to speak up. Share with your colleagues when you are emotionally harmed. Reach out for help from colleagues or specifically trained therapists when needed. Look out for your colleagues and ask them if they are okay, and press harder when you get the typical response of, "Yeah, I'm good." Consider asking: "Do you need help? Do you need to be heard or to vent? Do you need a hug?" Demand from your employer appropriate resources and specifically trained and qualified therapists who understand the unique mindset of those in this business. Teach those who are entering the field that it is a normal human response to feel something in times of human tragedy. Change the culture of not speaking up and sharing. Make it normal and part of the process to debrief after traumatic events, with all those involved. If it becomes acceptable to do all these things, then, in emergency services and in all of healthcare, it *will* be okay to say, "I am not okay."

WHAT IF!

REFERENCES

Bashore, Melvin L., and H. Dennis Tolley. "Mortality on the Mormon Trail, 1847–1868." *BYU Studies Quarterly* 53, no. 4 (2014): 109–123.

Brown, Mark. *Emergency!: True Stories from the Nation's ERs.* St. Martin's Paperbacks, 1997.

Davis, Matthew A., Benjamin A. Y. Cher, Christopher R. Friese, and J. P. W. Bynum. "Association of US Nurse and Physician Occupation with Risk of Suicide." *JAMA Psychiatry* 78, no. 6 (2021): 651–658. doi: 10.1001/jamapsychiatry.2021.0154

Vigil, Neil H., Samuel Beger, Kevin S. Gochenour, Weston H. Frazier, Tyler F. Vadeboncoeur, and Bentley J. Bobrow. "Suicide Among the Emergency Medical Systems Occupation in the United States." *Western Journal of Emergency Medicine* 22, no. 2 (2021): 326–332. doi: 10.5811/westjem.2020.10.48742

White, Ron. *They Call Me "Tater Salad."* Capitol Records, 2003.

Silent Trauma: The side of healthcare we don't talk about

Ziglar, Zig. A Checkup From The Neck Up. Nightingale-Conant, 1985.

ACKNOWLEDGEMENTS

A special shout-out to Bekah Ott. Her creativity is unmatched. She designed my book cover and offered more useful insight and encouragement than she realizes.

This book would still be just a file in my Google Drive were it not for two of my nieces, Kistie Adams and Kaylee Welker, doing editing, formatting, organizing, advising, publishing, and giving unwavering support. They are as talented as they are beautiful.

A very special thank-you to Sheila Anulao, the nurse on my cover, and a colleague I worked with side by side for years. Sheila encompasses everything I try to convey in this book. She taught me much about pediatric emergency nursing. Sheila left the ER and nearly all of nursing after many years of accumulated traumatic stress and one huge event. Thankfully, she is still in it as a pediatric and neonatal critical-care transport nurse. Thank you for sharing your story and heartache with me, and especially your journey to heal your moral injury. You are a rock star and the perfect example that it IS OKAY to say, "I am not okay."

To say my parents made me who I am is a profound understatement. I had the best upbringing anyone could wish for. My forever love to Jerry and Vickie Williamson, my dad and mom.

My greatest acknowledgement is reserved for the four human beings who are also my greatest accomplishment. In spite of my many poor decisions, they have all become terrific adults. For my children, I always wanted them to be kind and honest. In this success, I take great comfort. My Ashlie Bear, Scooter (Brian II), Z-Man (Zach), and my sweet Becca Boo. Also, the grandchildren they have given me so far: Loie, Trey (Brian III), Lincoln, Chapman, ZoraLyn, and Sophie.

ABOUT THE AUTHOR

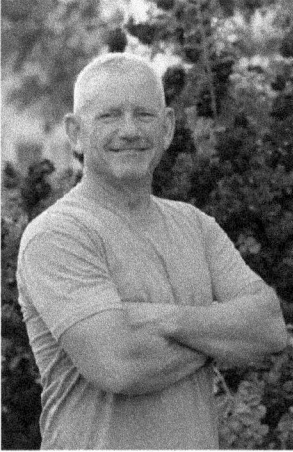

Brian has spent the majority of his career working in southern California's major acute care hospitals, trauma centers, and academic university medical centers. He also spent his time as a flight nurse in the southwestern United States. Brian is a certified legal nurse consultant who works with malpractice attorneys for both plaintiffs and defendants. Brian is also a testifying expert witness in emergency, critical care, and prehospital cases. He speaks on traumatic stress to nursing and provider groups, first responders, and law enforcement. He speaks to the leadership of these groups on the recognition of stress and the resource options for their staff. He is a content expert for PTSD, moral injury, traumatic stress, and burnout. He continues to work in critical care transport. Brian resides in Kanab, Utah. and enjoys being a granddad and spending time with his family, playing the guitar, and getting a little mud on the tires of his Jeep.

www.ingramcontent.com/pod-product-compliance
Lightning Source LLC
Chambersburg PA
CBHW052124270326
41930CB00012B/2749